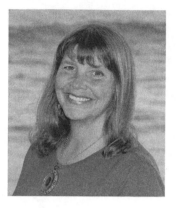

Lynne Cox was born in Boston, Massachusetts, and grew up in Los Alamitos, California, where she presently lives. She has held open water swimming records all over the world, including, first at age fifteen, twice setting the record for the fastest crossing of the English Channel, for men or women. Cox was a member of the first group of teenagers to cross the Catalina Channel in California. She has swum the twelve-mile Øresund and the Kattegat, both between Denmark and Sweden. Cox was the first woman to swim across the Cook Strait in New Zealand, and the first person to swim across the Strait of Magellan in Chile, the Beagle Channel between Argentina and Chile, Lake Baikal in Russia, and around the Cape of Good Hope in South Africa. In 1987 Cox crossed the Bering Strait from Alaska to the Soviet Union, and in 2002 swam more than a mile in the 31-degree Fahrenheit (0.5-degree Celsius) waters off Antarctica. Cox has been inducted into the International Swimming Hall of Fame. She is the author of *Swimming to Antarctica*, *Grayson*, and *South with the Sun*. Her articles have appeared in many publications, among them *The New Yorker* and the *Los Angeles Times Magazine*.

ALSO BY LYNNE COX

Grayson

South with the Sun

Swimming to Antarctica

Open Water Swimming Manual

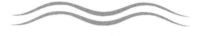

Open Water Swimming Manual

*An Expert's Survival Guide for Triathletes
and Open Water Swimmers*

LYNNE COX

Vintage Books
A Division of Random House, Inc.
New York

A VINTAGE ORIGINAL, JULY 2013

Charts and slides courtesy of the United States Navy SEALs

Library of Congress Cataloging-in-Publication Data:
Cox, Lynne.
Open water swimming manual : an expert's survival guide for
triathletes and open water swimmers / Lynne Cox.
pages cm
Includes index.
ISBN 978-0-345-80609-3 (pbk.)—ISBN 978-0-345-80610-9 (ebook)
1. Long distance swimming—Training.   I. Title.
GV838.53.L65C69 2013
797.2'1071—dc23   2013006165

Illustrations created by Estelle Cox
Author photograph © Ann Chatillon

www.vintagebooks.com

Printed in the United States of America
10   9   8   7   6   5   4   3

To the Cadre

Excellence is an art won by training and habituation.

—Aristotle

Contents

PART TWO: BEGINNING AND INTERMEDIATE SWIMMERS

PART THREE: INTERMEDIATE AND ADVANCED SWIMMERS

Introduction

The extreme is more accessible than ever before. People who never dreamed of venturing outside swimming pools, gyms, and manicured fields are venturing into the open water. They are no longer content to swim mega-laps in the swimming pool. They want to experience something new and more exciting. They want to push themselves as far as their arms will carry them and grow physically and mentally stronger. They want to feel what it's like to dream big, train hard, reach far, and, through the course of these experiences, explore the bounds of their inner and outer worlds.

Many people are entering the open water as a healthy way of escaping the constant noise and distractions of the world. They are slipping away from their computers, cell phones, and the barrage of daily information, and immersing themselves in clear blue and emerald-green waters, where they can think, meditate, and dream.

My primary reason for writing this book is to help people of all ages who are swimming or want to swim in the open water. I wrote it for people who already know how to swim and who are strong and competent swimmers; who have a background in competitive swimming; or who have experienced open water swimming with masters swimming groups, are triathletes, or have participated in junior lifeguard programs or are beach lifeguards.

I wanted to share my love of open water swimming with people who enjoy the feeling of being in the water and are eager to try new experiences and challenges. Also, for people who like to read about the outdoors, adventure, and nature, I wanted to provide a sense of what it's like to swim in the open water and across channels. It's fascinating to read other people's journeys and learn the lessons that they impart through their stories.

A large part of the manual is focused on our need to respect the power and unpredictability of the open water and of nature; to understand that safety is extremely important. Having qualified and knowledgeable support people and reliable watercraft are essential for open water swimming.

This is a manual for swimmers and triathletes who want to learn specific swimming skills and techniques for swimming in the open water. It will teach you special stroke mechanics that will help you in the swimming pool and in the open water. It also includes specific drills that will help you swim more efficiently and safely in the open water. I've provided training ideas and swim site suggestions. It includes information about ways to find open water swimming and triathlon coaches as well as contact information for associations that support channel swims.

The manual is divided into sections for beginning, intermediate, and advanced open water swimmers. The information presented here is fluid, there is overlap, and the topics are all interconnected. What applies to a beginning open water swimmer also applies to intermediate and advanced swimmers. For example, the steps a beginning open water swimmer would take to select a safe swimming area are the same methods an intermediate or advanced open water swimmer would use.

The sources of information for this manual include world experts: U.S. Navy SEALs; scientists who specialize in the marine environment; physicians who specialize in wilderness medicine, internal medicine, emergency medicine, dermatology, and other medical experts; the National Oceanic and Atmospheric Administration; the U.S. Coast Guard; current beach lifeguards, the American Lifeguard Association, and the United States Lifeguard Association; and other elite watermen and -women.

This book features open water swimming experiences and anecdotes from some of the best open water swimmers in the world. There are also stories about new open water swimmers and insights from triathletes who are currently training and competing at all levels of triathlon.

This manual will help open water swimmers learn how to break down their training into small segments and build upon their experiences, so that they can enjoy the feeling of getting stronger, more competent, more confident, and go as far as their bodies and minds enable them to go.

Just as U.S. Navy SEAL trainees use manuals to learn information pertinent to becoming U.S. Navy SEALs, they must also work with elite SEAL instructors who help them reach the high goal of becoming a SEAL (see Sources for website address; page 299). Similarly, this manual will give you the background knowledge to help you swim in the open water, but like the SEAL trainees, you need to train and to work with knowledgeable and qualified open water swimming coaches and/or triathlete coaches, or experienced and successful open water swimmers who can watch you swim on a daily basis, help you keep track of your progress, and help you improve. Although open water swimming is thought of as a solo sport, to really excel, you rely upon a team to help you achieve your goals. And if you train with a group, you may find that it's even more fun: a place where you give and gain inspiration and have longtime friendships.

At this time, a directory for open water swimming coaches does not exist, but there are well-established open water swim clubs and open water swimmers who provide a way to network and find a coach to help with your open water swimming. See Chapter 3 for guidelines for finding a coach and a team or club in your area.

When swimmers enter the open water, they begin their own water journeys. They are no longer swimming in a controlled area; they are entering a wild world where everything is constantly changing. Heraclites, the Greek philosopher, wrote, "You cannot step in the same river twice."

You will also discover that you cannot swim in the same river twice, and that is what makes the sport of open water swimming so exciting. Each swim is different—the way the water feels, the way it looks, the way you feel when you move through it. Each swim provides a different, often fascinating and sometimes life-altering experience.

You will find that as you spend more time in the open water, the experience becomes addictive in a good way, often a highlight of your day. Enjoy the water, time with friends, time to gain strength, and time to float and think and dream of near and distant horizons.

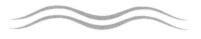

Open Water Swimming Manual

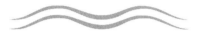

PART ONE

How to Begin

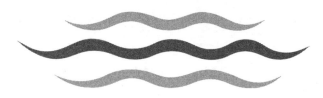

Chapter 1

Beginnings

ALLURE OF THE OPEN WATER

Oceans, lakes, rivers, ponds, and streams are some of the most beautiful places on earth to swim. Nothing compares with breaking free from the confines of a swimming pool and swimming in salty or sweet waters, as far as your arms will carry you. You are immediately lifted by the water, bounced by the waves, and massaged by the movement of your body through the water.

You feel sunshine warming your back, see shafts of sunlight illuminate the water below, hear the song of the wind and the waves, and as you swim, you hear the rhythms of your hands and feet as they catch and move water. You hear the music of your body and your breath as the wind, current, swell, and tide change, and the sounds of your body changing with it. You are immersed in this water song, and each day it is different.

Each day is a great adventure. You never know what you will experience until you get in and swim.

For forty years I have swum in the open water. At age fourteen I swam across the Catalina Channel and, at age fifteen, broke the men's and women's world records for the English Channel. Since then, I've completed sixty challenging open water swims—some were world-record swims, others were firsts, and all offered unique, exciting, and interesting challenges.

The sport of open water swimming is exploding like jogging did in the 1970s in the United States and Britain. There are more than nine hundred competitive open water swims across the United States throughout the year. There is a booming business in swim travel, in which swimmers travel to beautiful and exotic places like Greece, Turkey, and the Caribbean and participate in open water camps and swim along shore, between islands, and across straits.

The reason for this phenomenal growth in the sport may be because triathlon and open water swimming have gained Olympic status, since 2000 and 2008, respectively. According to the Sporting Goods Manufacturers Association (SGMA), an estimated 2.3 million people completed a triathlon in 2010, an increase of 55 percent from the year before, and the New York Triathlon sold out in eleven minutes despite an entry fee of just shy of nine hundred dollars (see Sources for more information; page 299).

Thomas Johnson, former president and current open water swim director of the Triathlon Club of San Diego (see Sources for website address; page 299), has watched this amazing growth and was involved with organizing the 2012 ITU World Triathlon San Diego, which served as the second qualifier for the 2012 U.S. Olympic Triathlon team. He predicted that the sport would expand even more after the Olympic qualifying event and Olympic Games.

John Martin, the communications and media relations manager at USA Triathlon, said there were 122,388 USA Triathlon members in 2000, and by 2012 there were 636,335 members. Martin said:

There are many reasons such as: society's interest in fitness and living a healthy lifestyle, the growth of the number of total races across the country, making events easier to get to, the growth in the number of the more accessible shorter sprint distance races, which made the sport more accessible to those with fewer hours to train each week, growth in the 30–49 age groups who are looking for varied outlets for fitness, an increase in the number of USA Triathlon clubs, which fosters a community concept for men and especially women who enjoy the group training and support atmosphere, an increase in resources (websites, books, magazines) that provide assistance/education in getting started, growth in multisport shops and triathlon-specific training and racing gear, marketing and communications efforts of USA Triathlon, the growth in the number of USA Triathlon certified coaches who are able to provide training plans and individual attention for athletes who need guidance and motivation, and USA Triathlon–sanctioned 4,300 multisport events in 2011.

This enormous expansion of triathlon has had a huge impact on the growth of open water because swimming is one of the races included in the triathlon. There has been a dramatic increase in media visibility and interest in both triathlon and open water swimming. Young swimmers are also participating in the sport, especially those who have been involved in junior lifeguard programs. Some university and college swimming coaches are incorporating open water swims during long-distance winter training sessions, to give the athletes a break from swimming thousands of mind-numbing meters in the pool. The swimmers are enjoying the challenge of swimming in the wild blue waters. Young and older swimmers who have spent years of their lives swimming back and forth in pools are reading books and magazines about open water swimming and triathlons and are inspired to swim in untamed water. They want to train, set open water swimming goals, and discover ways to make the extreme environment of the open water accessible for themselves.

Last year there were record numbers of people swimming the English Channel (between England and Europe) and the Catalina Channel (between Catalina Island and the mainland of California). The sport has become so popular that British television now broadcasts open water swims during prime time.

What most athletes don't realize is that open water swimming is a high-risk sport. This lack of awareness became very apparent to me on three separate occasions. The first occurred when a swimming friend in Laguna Beach, California, invited me to join him for an early dip. The fog was rolling in rapidly, reducing visibility to three hundred yards. We decided to swim only one hundred yards out to a buoy and then back in, because the fog was growing thicker, and we knew there was a chance of getting lost, even close to shore.

We met four triathletes, two men who had trained in the area a few times and two women who had never swum off that beach. They were planning to swim out to the buoy, parallel the shore, and swim toward cliffs about a half mile and back. One of the women asked if I would join them, and I said I didn't think it was safe.

They were wearing wet suits and dark caps, and they set off into a rolling wall of fog that quickly erased the sounds of their strokes and consumed them. Had they considered what would happen to them if the fog suddenly grew thicker; what they would do if they became separated or disoriented? Did they know how to find their way back to shore? Did they realize that they were completely invisible in the fog? Did they realize boaters and Jet Skiers wouldn't be able to see them and could easily run over them? They were oblivious to the risk they had taken or their responsibility to ensure the safety of their group. They were lucky they made it back without a problem.

A few weeks later, a friend who was just learning how to swim in the ocean was swimming parallel to shore outside the surf line. He had completed his workout and was turning in to the beach to swim to shore.

He forgot that he needed to look back to check the surf conditions. He was completely unaware that the dark blue long bump in the ocean was a wave growing behind him. He did not realize that this wave was a shore break. He suddenly felt the wave rapidly lifting him higher and higher and higher, tipping him forward and launching him into the air. He felt himself falling and the water rushing around him and suddenly pounding him into the beach.

He closed his eyes and felt himself flipping over the falls as tons of water crashed onto his body. He spun around and tried to find air, but the white water filled with sand was holding him under. His head finally broke the surface for a moment, and he gasped for a breath and tried to get his feet under him, but another wave, just as large, crashed on him and bounced him like a basketball on the beach.

He was submerged for what seemed like forever, but at last he planted his feet, stood up, and stumbled toward shore. The rip created by the backwash dragged him backward into the path of the approaching wave.

For the first time, he glanced over his shoulder and saw the next wave cresting. He leaned forward and, using his core strength, fought the backwash, pushed hard into the sand with feet, and staggered out of the water, coughing, his goggles twisted on his head, sand streaming down his face, shoulders, chest, sides, and filling his swimsuit. He looked up at his friends who had run down the beach to help him. He waved and smiled sheepishly and said he was okay. He understood that he could have been severely hurt in the shore break.

Shortly after that, I watched another swimmer, in his midforties, swimming off Seal Beach, California. He was breathing only on the right side of his body, so he was completely blind on the left. Because of this breathing pattern, he pulled stronger with his right arm than with his left. He had no spatial awareness, no sense of ocean navigation, and he could not see that he was swimming right into an area of heavy boating traffic. He had no idea that he was putting himself in danger. He was okay once he reached shore.

It was because of these events and many others that I realized there needed to be a book for all levels of open water swimmers, including those of us who have been swimming in the open water for years but still have so much to learn.

Scientists, physicians, lifeguards, and other experts offered to provide key information to help swimmers become more aware of the open water environment and to know how to handle themselves in the water.

EXPERT SOURCES AND CREDENTIALS

Even though I'd completed swims in remote parts of the world and I'd worked with various navies and coast guards to achieve my goals, I knew that there was so much more to know about seamanship, risk management, and other topics connected to open water swimming.

A friend in the United States Air Force offered to put me in touch with the U.S. Navy SEALs. The SEALs are members of the United States Naval Special Warfare unit, or NSW, who are trained for unconventional warfare; "SEAL" is an acronym for "sea, air, and land." NSW is the agency that provides units to conduct maritime special operations, since the SEALs are America's elite maritime force. They know more about operational risk management than anyone; they are the experts in assessing, reducing, and mitigating risks. They have established protocols that they abide by to ensure safety. They are experts in seamanship, can work in teams, and know how to survive in the wildest ocean conditions.

The SEALs welcomed me to their base in Coronado, California, to observe their sessions with the trainees, instructors, and officers, to see the best in the world train, to

understand the way the elite force implements safety measures, and to observe how everything is done in a completely
professional way.

I was allowed to sit in during the instructors' discussions about the trainees, which enabled me to understand
the amount of planning, discussion, and attention to detail
that goes into each training evolution, or session. They discussed everything in precise detail: how to initiate drills
and exercises, how long each one will last, how to ensure
the trainees' safety, how often the trainees hydrate, how
frequently the metal scuba tanks sitting in the hot sun are
cooled to prevent the trainees from being burned. They
reviewed how they would inspect each trainee, what errors
to check for, and the number of push-ups trainees would do
if they made a mistake. They also let me see the high-risk
documentation that ensured the trainees' safety. Equally
important, the SEALs let me see the level of qualification required by every instructor who supervises a training event, whether it's something as simple as a run or as
complex as a dive.

The senior SEAL who contributed so much invaluable
information, anecdotal stories, and guidance cannot be
named because he is on active duty, so I will refer to him
as L. Tadeus. His credentials are tremendously impressive.
He enlisted in the U.S. Navy, earned his commission as an
officer, and spent fourteen years working in the U.S. Navy
SEAL teams—eight years operational and six years in a
high-risk training capacity, supervising almost every type
of high-risk maritime training conducted by Special Operations Forces (SOF). He has spent three years specifically
conducting physical training events, from 2-mile to 5.5-
mile (3.2-kilometer to 8.8-kilometer) swims and 4-mile
(6.4-kilometer) runs. He is a Combatant Dive Training
subject matter expert; Command Diving Officer and Diving Supervisor; Submersible Pilot/Navigator; and Military
Small Craft Operator. The SEAL is trained in all levels of
Operational Risk Management, is a Military Master Train-

ing Specialist (MTS) 9502 NEC, and has earned numerous civilian maritime certifications, up to and including two-hundred-ton boats, and is a certified Captain Near Coastal (International Yacht Training [IYT]).

Among L. Tadeus's many training credentials is an additional qualification that made a huge difference to this manual. Like other senior SEALs, he has analyzed and investigated accidents that occurred during training. When he was not the actual Investigating Officer, he closely followed safety mishap investigations in cooperation with his Command Safety Manager to ensure that appropriate lessons were learned, and he institutionalized those lessons within the training curriculum so that no one would have to relearn them the hard way. He offered me many helpful illustrations of dangerous swim-training scenarios. He provided recommendations for finding support boats and people, equipment, and methods for incorporating risk management into open water swimming. He also gave me pearls of wisdom that he earned and learned through challenging experiences as a SEAL, an instructor, and a leader. He shared his knowledge generously to help open water swimmers swim safely and to help them achieve their worthy goals.

Rick Knepper also provided invaluable information. Rick is a sixty-three-year-old retired Navy SEAL Master Chief who has spent the past forty-five years with the Naval Special Warfare community, both for active duty and civil service. He has spent approximately thirty years working within the SEAL schoolhouse, with extensive time training SEAL candidates in all fundamental aquatic skills and surface swimming for ocean swims up to five and a half nautical miles. Additionally, he has been an aquatics trainer for numerous instructors' staffs over the years and continues to fulfill this need when required. He has revised and designed various aquatic programs with the SEAL training pipeline and has served as an aquatics consultant with other navy organizations. For the past twenty-five years, Rick has been swimming open water marathons. At the age of fifty, he completed the Catalina Channel crossing and a local twenty-four-mile sanctioned solo swim off San Diego. He is currently training for a thirty-six-mile (57.9-kilometer) swim scheduled in 2013 off Coronado Island.

His routine conditioning includes various open water training swims, with several between fourteen and sixteen miles and occasionally up to twenty miles (32.1 kilometers). A purist, he swims year-round off San Diego without a wet suit, just a cap, goggles, and a swimsuit. He has served as the safety coordinator on several twelve-mile (19.3-kilometer) swims and supported other open water swimmers with their training and event goals. He contributed insights and suggestions from many years of experience as a SEAL and as an instructor.

Visiting the SEAL base gave me the invaluable opportunity to watch the best maritime special force unit in the world work with their trainees.

On a cool morning in March 2010 at the SEAL training base in San Diego, California, Mark James, a SEAL instructor, invited me to join him and the trainees in a classroom for a briefing before the trainees entered the water. The briefing would inform the trainees what they'd be doing during their training session and would answer any questions before they entered the water.

Mark James referred to a diagram of the swim course, beautifully drawn on a large chalkboard. Point by point, he discussed the swim. He told the trainees the water temperature was 58 degrees F (14.4 degrees C), that the surf was negligible but the current to the north was strong. They would be swimming parallel to the shore to the north for a nautical mile—two thousand yards. They would get a strong current assistance to north, and they would need to work on their navigation skills to hold a straight line to the buoy. Once they reached the buoy, they would swim counterclockwise around the buoy and then back to the base.

This would be a timed swim, and they were instructed to stay within six feet of their swim buddy, who was another trainee. They watched out for each other.

Medical responders in a truck onshore had put a number of safety mechanisms in place, so all the trainees had to do was focus on their training. Mark James would be riding a Jet Ski, and there would be qualified instructors in an escort boat alongside the swimmers. There would also be an emergency response team on the beach, keeping pace with the swim the whole time. At some point during the swim, the trainees would practice an emergency rescue drill. One swimmer would be selected to simulate a swimmer in distress. The crew on the support boat would convey to the medical responders onshore, in a truck, that there was an emergency situation and then signal everyone involved in the training session by using a smoke signal, or pulling smoke. The people in operations who monitored all the training were reminded of the rescue drill and the fact that a trainee would be pulling smoke.

When the boat and Jet Ski were in place, an instructor on the beach started the SEAL trainees. Outfitted in wet suits, the trainees quickly entered the rusty-red Pacific off Coronado Island, dove under small swells, and swam north using the special combat swimmer's stroke, a modified sidestroke, that enabled them to reduce their splash in the water and make them far less visible than freestyle.

The group quickly became a long line of swimmers moving parallel to shore. The escort boat and Jet Ski support crew watched to make sure they all made it around the buoy. As they swam quickly and efficiently, the responders in trucks monitored what was happening. All their focus was on the trainees.

When the majority of the swimmers had nearly reached the finish of the swim, the rescue drill was initiated, with the "stricken" trainee's buddy pulling smoke. A white trail of smoke rose like a white line above the water and signaled the men in the safety boat that a trainee was in trouble. The SEAL instructor on the Jet Ski responded immediately. He moved carefully around the swimmers, pulled up beside the swimmer who needed to be rescued, and with the help of one other swimmer, he helped place the stricken trainee on a rescue sled. The trainees who noticed the smoke shouted to the other swimmers to muster, meaning they needed to get out of the water quickly and go to a designated area where two other instructors could check their names off a list to account for everyone.

Meanwhile, the Jet Skier came ashore through the surf and met the emergency response team at the water's edge. They placed the victim on a spine board, settled him in the truck, and transported him to the medical clinic onsite. The team timed the drill and was pleased with the rapid response. After the training session, the instructors debriefed, or discussed, the swim with the trainees and went over questions. It was amazing to observe how the best in the world train and how they put safety mechanisms in place. So much that is both seen and unseen goes into planning a training session, so that all the trainees have to worry about is performing.

It takes a certain kind of swimmer to want to venture beyond the cement walls and enter a world that is as different from Earth as space. It takes someone who is looking for something more challenging, that is constantly changing, that makes her think about how she's being affected by the forces of nature, and how she needs to use physical strength and mind to move through the open water.

It is a dramatic, exciting, and thrilling world, but in order to swim in the open water, you need to be a strong, competent swimmer who can evaluate risks, know how to mitigate them, and decide when it is safe to swim. It helps a lot if you have swum on competitive teams or in masters programs, participated in junior lifeguard programs, competed in triathlons, or played water polo. That is not to say other athletes should not swim in the open water, but they need to reach a certain level of competency before they venture into the surf, current, and waves.

As in every sport, you need to begin with the proper equipment.

Chapter 2

Equipment

THE SWIMSUIT

For most swimmers, the essential apparel is a swimsuit. A number of swimsuit manufacturers have designed suits that work well for open water swimming; these include, in alphabetical order, Adidas, AgonSwim, Arena, Nike, Speedo, and TYR. As with running shoes, there are a variety of swimsuits to choose from; swimsuits are cut, sewn, and fit differently, and they are available in different materials. It is worth taking the time to find a style that fits your body and a fabric that works best for you.

The fabric matters. Some swimmers want a swimsuit that is stretchy, some want one that is warmer, and some want a suit that is durable. Swimsuits are available in three basic fabrics: Lycra, polyester, and spandex, as well as blends of these fabrics. The amount of polyester and spandex and whether the fabrics are knitted or woven make the difference in the way the fabrics feel.

Lycra swimsuits are the thinnest and have the most stretch. Swimming in a Lycra swimsuit feels almost as if you're wearing nothing. The Lycra clings to and moves with your body. The fabric allows you to feel the water.

Polyester and polyester/spandex blends are thicker,

more durable, a bit warmer, and less revealing than Lycra. They are also heavier and offer more resistance in the water. That's why many pool swimmers train in heavier nylon or polyester blends and wear lighter Lycra swimsuits for competitions. Lycra swimsuits fade, and the material breaks down more quickly than polyester blends, but in the chlorine-free open water, all swimsuit fabrics will have longer lives.

The most important consideration when selecting a swimsuit is fit. If a running shoe doesn't fit well, you'll get blisters; if a swimsuit doesn't fit well, it will chafe. Salt water is very abrasive, and if you're swimming considerable distances in the ocean, you will be chafed. For women, the areas that chafe the most are along the seams of the suit, around the top of the suit, under the arms, and around the leg holes. For men, swimsuits chafe along the seams, around the top of the suit, and around the leg holes. Unfortunately, swimsuit manufacturers construct swimsuits with the seams on the underside of the suit instead of on the outside.

When Laura, my younger sister, and I began open water swimming—long before the term was used to describe long-distance ocean or freshwater swimming—we wore tough nylon swimsuits. The seams were thick and abrasive, and after long workouts, the seams rubbed us red and raw; eventually, the seams cut into our skin. Clothes and Band-Aids stuck to the cuts, and when we changed clothes, we gently peeled off the scabs and often bled.

Our father, a physician, was very concerned about infection; our mother, an artist who was very good at sewing, suggested that we invert our swimsuits. That way, the seams would be on the outside of the swimsuit and not up against our skin. Her idea considerably reduced chafing along the swimsuit seams, but we were swimming long distances, and the swimsuits still chafed.

Our mother had another solution. She took a one-inch-wide elastic strip used to make waistbands for pants, measured around Laura's waist and around mine, and sewed the ends of the waistbands together and gave one to each of us. We put on our swimsuits, pulled the waistbands over our heads to our waists, and when we went swimming and reached deep water, we pulled off our swimsuit straps and let the top part of the swimsuit drop down to our waists. The elastic band kept the swimsuit from falling off, and when we completed our workouts, we put the top of our swimsuit back on and swam in to shore.

Today swimsuits are made from softer materials, but they still chafe. Recently, a friend in San Diego was swimming long distances in La Jolla and was getting chafed badly by her swimsuit. She made the elastic waistband and used our solution.

SWIMSUIT CARE

Chlorine bleaches in swimming pools quickly break down swimsuit fabrics. Swimsuits used in the open water have much longer lives. In either case, caring for your swimsuits will extend their lives.

~ Hand-wash the swimsuit.
~ Gently wring the water out of the swimsuit.
~ Hang-dry inside the shower, or place it where it can drip-dry.
~ While the sunshine will dry a swimsuit faster than inside the house, sunlight fades and breaks down the swimsuit fabrics.
~ Avoid putting swimsuits in the dryer. High heat cooks the material, especially Lycra, and it will have a very short life.

Many people who do double workouts have a couple of suits, since most swimmers don't like to put on a wet swimsuit for the second workout. But if you have only one, you can wash your swimsuit with soap and water while you're in the shower, to save time; when you're done, wrap your swimsuit in a towel to absorb the moisture, then hang it to dry.

CHAFING

In addition to the chafing problems described above, men can have chafing caused by facial hair. A beard or even the short stubble of a day's hair growth can chafe the shoulders and area around the neck until they are raw. Sometimes the movement of the arms and turning the head causes chafing. This also happens to the SEAL trainees on their long-distance swims. One friend who swims long distances in the open water was chafed so much around his neck from one day's growth that a stranger stopped him and asked if he'd tried to hang himself!

Another major area of chafing for men and women is under the arms. After long open water swims, skin is often rubbed raw under the arms. Women's swimsuits also chafe a lot along the sides and may cut into the sides of the breasts.

SKIN LUBRICATION PRODUCTS

When swimmers first swam across the English Channel, they used black axle grease to coat their bodies, for warmth and to reduce chafing. Because of problems with chafing, there were top female open water swimmers in the 1920s and '30s who swam naked. Today there are women who wear two-piece swimsuits until they get into the water, and then they ditch their tops, hand them over to their escort paddlers, and when they finish their workout, they put the tops back on and swim ashore.

Lanolin, Vaseline, Bag Balm, and BodyGlide are skin lubricants that have been used for years by open water swimmers. Some swimmers make their own mixture of lubricants. All of them help reduce chafing. When applying them to your skin, make sure that you wear rubber gloves or surgical gloves before smearing your skin with the lubricants. This will prevent the lubricant from sticking to your fingers and smearing your goggles. There's nothing worse than looking out through lubricant-smeared goggles for hours on end not being able to see clearly during the swim. More than annoying, though, is a swimmer's inability to see the escort boat and support crew. You need to be visually connected to both throughout the swim and be alert for any sign of danger. Little things like having clear goggles make the difference between having an enjoyable swim and a very frustrating one.

Lanolin, Vaseline, and body glide lubricants, and mixtures of these three, are used most by open water swimmers, and all have advantages and disadvantages.

Lanolin

Lanolin is also known as wool wax or wool grease. Sheep's glands secrete this yellow waxy substance to help them shed water from their woolly coats. Lanolin also protects their coats and skin from harsh dry and cold environments.

For years lanolin has been used in skin care products to protect, moisturize, and beautify the skin. Certain breeds of sheep produce large amounts of lanolin. Men and women in countries like New Zealand and Australia, who work on sheep stations and shear hundreds of sheep, not only have strong hands from shearing and holding down the sheep; they have super-soft hands from the lanolin.

Once the wool is harvested, it is pressed between rollers to extract the lanolin. For years English Channel swimmers have used lanolin to protect their skin, reduce chafing, and keep them warm. According to William Keatinge, MD, one of the world's experts on hypothermia, there is no real evidence that lanolin helps a swimmer retain a significant amount of body heat, although it does help to reduce chafing and protect the skin.

At one time, lanolin was readily available at pharmacies worldwide, as it was often used as a compounding agent for skin care products, but it now has to be special-ordered from pharmacies in England or the United States. Swimmers who use lanolin in the English Channel can find chemists in Folkestone and Dover who sell the product.

The type of lanolin open swimmers use is a gooey substance that is a light to medium yellow and feels like marshmallow cream. It is available in a variety of thicknesses. Some lanolin is so thick that it is difficult to apply. Most pharmacists in Dover and Folkestone know what kind of lanolin swimmers require, but it helps to tell them that it should be easy to apply but thick enough to stay on for a long time

There are drawbacks to using lanolin. It smells greasy, sweet, and musty, like an old wet woolen sweater. Some swimmers don't mind the smell, but if you're swimming beside a fishing boat, the odor of dead fish wafting by on the breeze coupled with the heavy smell of diesel fumes from the boat's engines that you get whiffs of now and then, there is a good possibility that all these smells may make you queasy. Over time, this irritant may reduce your capability.

The other major consideration is that lanolin is a substance rendered from an animal by-product. The scent of sheep in the water may attract the wrong crowd—large fish with teeth or marine mammals may mistake a swimmer for food.

Lanolin usually stays on a swimmer's body so well that it can be difficult to remove in the shower or bathtub after finishing the swim. Kevin Murphy, one of the greatest

British open water swimmers, advised me after my first English Channel swim to use liquid dishwashing detergent to cut through the lanolin. It required half a bottle. This works for Vaseline and BodyGlide as well, though they can also be removed with shampoo or skin soap, which may be gentler on the skin.

Aquaphor

Recently, a friend of mine completed a fifteen-hour swim across the San Pedro Channel and said that he used a thick coat of Aquaphor ointment in the areas that chafed. He said it worked very well and stayed on through the swim.

Aquaphor is a product that Dr. Laura King, a dermatologist and a member of my support crew, has recommended for chapped lips and for too much sun and saltwater exposure. The Aquaphor helps the skin retain moisture and helps it heal.

Alternative Lubricants

Another solution for chafing came from my friend Greg Miller, who is a national champion cyclist. He competed in the Race Across America (RAAM) when it first began in 1982, racing from the Santa Monica Pier in Los Angeles to the Empire State Building in New York City. He also trained with the professional Belgian cycling team with the idea that he would go pro.

Greg said that they cycled for up to eight hours a day in all kinds of conditions, including ice and snow, and during the long rides, they experienced real problems with chafing. The Belgian team's solution was to place large beefsteaks inside their cycling shorts and between their butts and the bicycle saddles. Greg said the bicycle seat tenderized the steaks instead of their backsides. He said it was awfully messy, but it literally saved their butts.

While this tactic worked well for the cyclists, swimming with steaks in your swimsuit could attract the big fish. But you can always learn something from top competitors in other sports. Friends who still compete in Race Across America have discovered the lubrication qualities of Desitin, an ointment used primarily to prevent diaper rash. The RAAM cyclists use large amounts of the ointment on their butts and other areas that chafe. Though they sweat a lot during their races, they say the Desitin doesn't wash off. An added benefit is that it contains zinc, a compound that's been used as a sun block for years. You may find it helpful on long open water swims.

Which lubricant you use is a highly personal choice. Keep the following things in mind when deciding:

~ During your training sessions, test the various lubricants and see what will work best for you. If you don't want to be bothered by applying the lubricant with rubber gloves, either use your ring fingers to apply the lubricant, or make sure to wash your hands with soap and water. Otherwise, you will be looking through smeared goggles.

~ When applying these lubricants, make sure you don't get any on your face; if you do, it will get on your goggles. Use waterproof sunscreen on your face, but make sure you apply it above your eyebrows and around your goggle area; otherwise the sunscreen will drip into your eyes and will sting and make it difficult to see and swim.

~ Apply globs of lubricant to your skin to make sure it will stay for the entire swim. It is difficult to reapply during a swim, and the time it takes to do so will cause you to cool down. Be sure to apply enough for your swim.

~ Some swimmers prefer to cover all of their exposed skin and their swimsuits with the lubricant. Some swimmers apply the lubricant only to key points of friction along their bodies. Some male swimmers apply lubricant to all the unexposed areas beneath their swimsuits.

~ The best way to remove the lubricant is with soap and water during a warm to hot shower.

~ Lanolin is more adhering, and if you want to get it off quickly, dishwashing soap works best.

~ Soaps will dry out the skin. Dr. King recommends using body lotions after long swims to put moisture back into the skin. The swimsuit will also chafe less if your skin is moist.

TREATMENT FOR CHAFING

Whether your swimsuit chafes enough to make your skin red or so much that it cuts into your skin, there's a chance those spots can become infected. It's important to take care of the affected areas.

Dr. King advises doing the following:

~ Wash the area with soap and water to reduce the bacterial count.

~ Use Aquaphor, an over-the-counter cousin of Vaseline, that has been shown to have antimicrobial properties and is just as effective as Neosporin or bacitracin at helping to heal minor infections. Aquaphor has the benefit of very little to no risk of allergic contact dermatitis, whereas bacitracin is the most common contact allergen in the United States, followed closely by Neosporin.

SUNSCREEN PRODUCTS

Most people are aware that prolonged exposure to UVA and UVB rays from the sun damages the skin and may lead to skin cancer. Experts believe skin damage can be averted by using sunscreen.

Swimmers should use a waterproof sunscreen with an SPF of 30 or higher. No sunscreen is completely waterproof, so try a variety of sunscreens during workouts. Apply

> This was something I learned on my training swims in Lake Titicaca. At an altitude of 12,500 feet, and with the reflective element of the water, I got burned.

the sunscreen an hour before a workout or event so it has time to be absorbed into the skin. Reapply every hour if possible.

No sunscreen has been conclusively proven to stay on better than others, and there probably is no difference for open water swims versus non—open water, although salt water is abrasive and may cause sunscreen to come off faster than fresh water. The effects of the UVA and UVB are more dramatic at high altitude, and in the southern hemisphere, where the ozone layer is thinner. That makes it all the more important to reapply sunscreen regularly.

SUNBURN PREVENTION

Another way to prevent sunburn is to wear protective clothing, which can also be helpful in preventing seabather's eruption and swimmer's itch (see Chapter 13, pages 203 and 213). There are some shirts out there that don't balloon up in the water. But one of the problems with the sun-protective cloth is that it is tightly woven and hence pretty warm. These fabrics may also cause chafing.

SUNBURN TREATMENT

Dr. King advises the following treatment for sunburns:

~ It is best to act quickly, within a few hours of sun exposure. Aspirin is a very good anti-inflammatory and cuts down on sunburn reaction as well as being a painkiller.
~ Cortisone creams are soothing, too. The over-the-counter strength is pretty mild and won't be that effec-

tive, but the prescription-strength steroid (synonymous with "cortisone") creams are helpful when applied twice a day to burns. The more common generic names are fluocinonide 0.05% cream and clobetasol 0.05% cream.

~ In severe cases, oral cortisone (prednisone or a Medrol Dosepak) can be used.

~ If you have a severe burn, get professional medical attention.

GOGGLES

Goggles are essential for open water swimming. They enable a swimmer to see above and under the water. They reduce eye irritation from salt water and other elements. Like sunglasses, they reduce the glare on the water and enable the swimmer to see obstacles, such as boats and windsurfers. Some goggles with UVA and UVB protection can protect swimmers' eyes from the sun's harmful rays and reduce the chances of cataracts.

Speedo, TYR, Barracuda, Aqua Sphere, Jaguar, Wiley, FINIS, Cressi, Body Glove, Blue Seventy, Aqua World, and even Marvel and Disney make swimming goggles. They are available in a wide variety of styles, colors, sizes, and shapes. Swimming goggles must fit. If they leak, they will become a distraction and could affect the outcome of a long-distance swim.

Finding a pair of goggles is like selecting a pair of shoes. Some people like goggles that are very tiny and rest inside the eye orbit; some prefer that the goggle create a seal around the eyebrows and on the cheeks; others would rather wear a swim mask.

The best way to choose goggles is to go to a swimming supply or sports store and try them on. Hold the goggles up to your face until they create suction, but do not put the straps over your head. If the goggles stay on your face for about ten to twenty seconds, you have a good seal, and the goggles fit your face. No matter how stylish the goggles are, don't purchase them if they do not fit.

The straps are used to hold the goggles in place. If you are tightening your straps so much that the cups leave a deep imprint around your eyes and you look like a raccoon after a workout, you are pulling your straps too tight. If you are getting headaches from the goggles, you are probably wearing the straps too tight.

After you have adjusted the goggle straps so that they fit comfortably, move on to the nosepiece, which some brands allow you to adjust. If the nosepiece pinches, you have pulled it too tight. The nosepiece area should fit comfortably, and water should not leak in from either side of the nose. If it does, then you need to find a different pair of goggles. Some swim equipment manufacturers make smaller goggles to fit a woman's face, as well as goggles just for children.

The lens color is an important consideration. For open water swimming during daylight hours, I like smoked or darker-tinted goggles. The darkness cuts the glare. Many of my friends use red-, amber-, green-, or blue-tinted goggles.

Clear goggles do not reduce the glare. During a night swim, or in the early morning before the sun has risen, I usually wear clear goggles. Smoked goggles make everything very dark and reduce your ability to see at night.

One pair of goggles is usually all you need for a workout, but during a long open water swim, it is important to have three or four pairs of goggles in case the ones you're wearing leak. Test all of your goggles during your workouts to make sure they fit.

When trying a new set of goggles during a workout, I usually wear the pair that

Even if you're careful, it is easy to smear Vaseline, sunscreen, or lanolin on your goggles, and it is not fun swimming with restricted vision. I made that mistake on my first English Channel swim.

I know fits, and I either carry the test pair around my wrist or in the small of my back, under my suit, until I want to take them out and test them.

Usually, a swimmer will find a certain style of goggle that fits, like a favorite pair of shoes, and will stay with that style, but sometimes it is fun to try out new colors and shapes and see if they work for you.

The life of your goggles depends on how well you take care of them. Some swimmers have a favorite pair that lasts three or four years. To extend the life of your goggles, rinse them out in fresh water after you use them. If they came with a case, use it; it will reduce the chance of their getting scratched or broken.

> Goggles sometimes fog, making it difficult to see out of them. Licking the goggles is something that swimmers have done for years to clear the lenses.

SWIM CAPS

There are basically three types of swimming caps made from different material: Lycra, latex, and silicone. A swim cap has two important functions in open swimming: to keep the swimmer warm by reducing heat loss through the head; and to make the swimmer more visible when swimming. But don't count on any swim cap to keep your hair dry.

Lycra is a stretchy and breathable fabric, though it doesn't provide much insulation, and the fabric is not as bright in color as latex or silicone. I have tried Lycra swim caps during open water swimming, and I believe that latex or silicone swim caps are better choices. Latex caps fit the swimmer's head very well and grip on. They are a bit thinner than silicone swim caps, and they tend to pull your hair if not removed carefully.

While I've used all three types of swim caps over the years, I think silicone caps work the best. Some swimmers

Other Equipment: Fins and Paddles

Fins and paddles are good training tools in the swimming pool, but in the open water, they can give you a false sense of confidence. My preference is not to use them as a tool for open water swimming.

feel that they slide around their head somewhat, but I would rather adjust my swimming cap than have my hair torn. The silicone swim cap usually has a much longer life than the latex swim cap. It is somewhat more expensive than the latex, but it lasts longer, doesn't tear my hair, and better reduces the heat loss through my head. Expect to replace your swim cap once or twice a year.

I pick colors that the beach lifeguards along the California coast can see. Bright orange, bright yellow, and bright red are my choices for daylight swimming. Black, blue, green, and silver are not as visible in the ocean and are not good choices. During a night or early-morning swim before the sun rises, I usually wear a white or yellow swim cap.

WET SUITS

Many open water swimmers are purists; they wear only swimsuits, no wet suits. Their goal is to attempt and complete a swim under their own power. However, there are growing numbers of open water swimmers and triathletes who want to wear wet suits.

Bruce Jones, a longtime surfer who owns Bruce Jones Surfboards in Sunset Beach, California, has been fitting surfers with O'Neill wet suits for years. Surfing wet suits are generally thicker than wet suits meant for open water swimmers and triathletes, but for any of these water sports, there are some basic considerations when buying a suit.

Jones says that the three most important factors are fit, construction, and thickness. When he helps a person find a wet suit, he first checks the size chart supplied by the manufacturer and then has the individual try on the wet suit in the store. The wet suit cannot be loose; it needs to be a little tight, as it will soften up when you get into the water.

Wet suits trap a thin layer of water that warms up if you are moving and creating heat. Jones says if you aren't moving, you won't stay warm, unless you're in tropical waters. If you are swimming in cold water, he advises choosing a wet suit with glued and blind-stitched seams; otherwise the seams will leak. If you are swimming in warm to hot water, you need to get a wet suit that is flat-stitched. The flat-stitch has tiny needle holes along the seams and allows some water to enter the wet suit, which cools it down. Most surfers use wet suits that are two millimeters thick; most triathletes use wet suits that are half a millimeter to one millimeter thick.

Leonard Kurp, who owns the Tri-Pacific shop in Long Beach, California, is a triathlete who believes that the best manufacturers of wet suits for triathletes and open water swimmers are Aqua Sphere, Blue Seventy, Orca, Profile Design, TYR, and Zoot. "These triathlon wet suits are all about speed," says Kurp. There are many different types, and if you are going to use one in competition, check with the United States Triathlon Association and the United States Master Swimming or the organizing body to make sure the wet suit is legal for use during your competition.

It matters how the wet suit is designed and how it fits. When you are trying to figure out what kind of triathlon wet suit to purchase, Kurp advises looking for one designed for flexibility, buoyancy, and speed. Advances in Yamamoto neoprene—wet-suit material—allow for greater flexibility; also, it is a slicker material that enables you to move quickly through the water with less resistance.

When looking at a triathlon wet suit, you should be able to see buoyancy panels across the chest and around the arms, legs, and glutes. These panels are sewn together to create the wet suit, and this construction enables you to move in a less restricted way than if you were wearing a wet suit made for surfers. Make sure there is a knee flex panel, which allows you to kick freely, as well as silicone seals around the wrists to prevent the arms from filling up with water. These wet suits also provide some warmth, and they are useful in cool or warm waters, but it's important to note that in tropical waters, you can overheat.

If you are swimming long distances in a triathlon wet suit, there is a good chance that it will chafe. You may want to apply BodyGlide or Aquaphor to reduce chafing, but don't use Vaseline, as the petroleum jelly will break down the neoprene.

SWIM SKINS

Swim skins are an alternate to triathlete wet suits. Mike Orton, a competitive swimmer in college, a triathlete, and now a sales representative for Blue Seventy, says that swim skins were designed for triathletes swimming in warm waters, like off Kona, Hawaii. They are made of a slick, nearly paper-thin fabric, a blend of polyester and spandex that enables a swimmer to slip through the water. Swim skins were used at the Olympic Games in Beijing, and they created a lot of controversy. Many of the swimmers who wore the swim skins broke world records. Since then, swim skins have been illegal for USA Swimming and Olympic swimming competitions, but they are still being used in triathlon competitions.

There are many swimmers who are purists, who want to achieve their best unaided—which I agree with—but swim skins offer additional advantages: They can reduce the amount of UVA and UVB exposure, and they may provide a barrier to jellyfish stings.

As with wet suits, always try on your swim skin to make sure you'll feel comfortable swimming in it.

Chapter 3

Finding an Open Water Swimming Coach and Group

Do not begin open water swimming on your own. Find an open water swimming coach and a group to swim with. Rick Knepper, the SEAL instructor and open water swimmer, explains why there are strong reasons to find a coach/ mentor and a group of swimmers to train with.

Linking up with the right person or group will enable developing swimmers to work collaboratively to sort out and manage their development as an open water swimmer; the more experienced the coach or overall group is, the sooner they can identify what is going well and what has the potential to cause disaster.

Every swimmer needs to realize that he or she is "an experiment of one," and the more experienced swimmers helping to find a good training plan, the better; lessons learned are tough in the sport of long-distance ocean swimming.

Find people who are experienced open water swimmers and have completed events, coached others, and participated in helping others by supporting crew/paddler activities. They are good for lessons learned, advice, and help for training and event day. Knowing and being associated with qualified people can be useful when life's schedules require you to ask several different people to help with a swim as a swimming partner or a paddler.

Selecting a qualified open water swimming coach is critical. Laura, my sister, has coached for over twenty-five years at Alamo Area Aquatic Association in Texas. She was a starter on the United States National Water Polo team, swam in Division One nationals, was the first female lifeguard at Huntington State Beach in California, assistant-coached men's swimming and water polo at Washington and Lee University, and has spent years devising technical approaches to swimming efficiency. She has listened to all the great coaches in the United States, learned from them, and incorporated that into her own coaching. She suggests asking these questions in order to evaluate a coach:

~ What is the coach's background and knowledge base in regard to open water swimming?

~ Is this going to be someone you can absolutely trust? Ultimately, you may be trusting him or her with your life.

You can use two general approaches to evaluate the knowledge base of a potential coach. The first approach is to find someone who is a well-known open water swimmer and/or successful and reputable open water coach. Because not many people fit into this first category, you can evaluate a person's credentials and assess his or her experience with open water safety through established competitive swimming organizations. In the United States, these are USA Swimming, the American Swimming Coaches Association, the United States Lifesaving Association, and the American Lifeguard Association. Essential questions regarding credentials include:

~ Is this person a certified coach with the American Swimming Coaches Association? If so, what level has he achieved? (Level 1 is the lowest level of experience.)

~ Is she a certified coach with USA Swimming? This
certification requires CPR, first aid, and coaches' safety
certifications, and also requires passing criminal background checks. These are the minimal requirements for
a professional swimming coach.

~ Is he or she certified through the United States Lifesaving Association or the American Lifeguard Association?

When looking for an open water swimming coach, you
want someone with these basic certifications; plus, you
want the coach to have open water experience. This may
include beach lifeguarding, open water competitions, or
training from a reputable and successful open water swimming coach.

Evaluating whether you can trust a potential coach is
more difficult but essential. In order to achieve your goals,
you need to find a coach with whom you can build a bond
of mutual trust. When you are in the middle of a difficult
situation, you need to know that you can absolutely trust
and rely on this person, that he or she will help you find
your inner strength and resolve but also will not recklessly
lead you into harm's way by either stretching you beyond
your physical limits or leading you into hazardous waters.
Building trust is an iterative process that begins with effective communication. That is, the coach will define the first
step in a process, and the swimmer will execute that step.
Based on the outcome of the first step (success, failure, no
change), the coach will define the next step, the swimmer
will execute it, and so on.

If you can't communicate clearly and effectively with
the potential coach, then you are unlikely to develop a beneficial relationship. Watch him or her coach. Do you like
the person's style? Do you like how she communicates and
motivates her athletes? Do the swimmers like him or fear
him? Which style do you need as an athlete? Do the workouts
appear challenging and interesting and fun, or are they bor-
ing and lacking mental engagement? Does the coach only

tell the athletes what to do? For example, does the coach just say, "Swim ten reps of one hundred meters freestyle in two minutes"? Or does the coach interact with the swimmers, providing technical feedback and further instructions for correction? Remember, simply telling a swimmer what he's doing wrong isn't useful. The coach must state what is wrong and how to correct it, then follow up, informing the swimmer whether the correction was made.

Set up a meeting with the potential coach to determine if she or he is genuinely interested in helping you achieve your goals. As part of this meeting, you need to clearly state your goals; the coach should be able to provide a plan that will include a training regimen and a general outline toward achieving the goal. Both the coach and swimmer must understand that there is a process of developing goals, training toward short-term goals, achieving short-term goals, and refining training and revising intermediate milestones on the path to the main goal. Through this process, the coach and swimmer build trust—the coach in the swimmer's desire, commitment, and determination to achieve the goal; and the swimmer in the coach's ability to lead, motivate, and provide the opportunities that will build the mental and physical skills necessary to achieve the goal. Building trust is intertwined with the iterative training program. The bond of trust between swimmer and coach should strengthen during this process. If it doesn't, then this person may have been great at one stage in your development but may not be whom you need to take you forward.

FINDING SPECIFIC COACHES AND GROUPS

One way to find open water swimming coaches and clubs is to try contacting U.S. Masters Swimming or some of the clubs and teams that have a long tradition of open water swimming.

U.S. Masters Swimming has a list of coaches and a list of open water swimming seminars and open water swimming races. The organization is a very good resource, and if you are a member, you can receive *SWIMMER* magazine, which features all aspects of open water and masters swimming. Laura Hamel, the editor, also suggested checking out their website for more information about clubs, coaches, and news about open water swimming (see Sources for website address; page 299).

There are also clubs and swim teams around the world for open water swimming. Two of the most established in the United States, each with a history of nurturing all levels of open water swimmers, are the South End Rowing Club, established in 1873, and the Dolphin Club, established in 1877, each among the oldest athletic clubs west of the Mississippi. They are located in Aquatic Park, near Fisherman's Wharf in San Francisco. Though they share a common wall, and both have a long tradition of open water swimming and rowing, they have very different philosophies.

Dolphin Club members limit the range of their swims to the cove in front of the clubhouse in Aquatic Park unless they are participating in a special event. The South End Rowing Club has swims throughout the bay. For more advanced open water swimmers, the South End Rowing club conducts daily open water swims for club members, and they often invite competent swimmers to train with them.

To participate in the South End swims or Dolphin Club swims, you need to be a club member. Members from all over the country travel to San Francisco when they can in order to swim with their club. Both clubs welcome swimmers of all abilities. As Bill Wygant, the former president of the South End Rowing Club, says,

We are accommodating and welcoming to swimmers of all types—yes, even with wet suits—for club swims. We take care of everyone on club swims and then feed them breakfast. But for our longer swim program, that tolerance kind of disappears, and you need to be able to make the swim or go home. We are a place that asks you to measure your own capabilities and self-select out if you are not trained or ready for a swim. On our longer swim program, when we say, "Get in the water," we don't want a lot of discussion about it. Just go, and we expect you to finish the swim. If not, we just stack you in the Zodiac and hope for the best. This is much different than the Dolphin Club. We like it that way.

Both clubs are great places to swim. They have an enormous wealth of knowledge based on more than one hundred years of swimming in the bay, and on accumulation of information from daily experiences of swimmers from both clubs. They also consult and work with the U.S. Coast Guard in San Francisco. The swims give their members the opportunity to swim in cool and cold water, in areas where there are very strong tides, currents, and wind. Conditions are similar to what swimmers experience on the English Channel and the Catalina Channel crossings, making the bay a great place to train for serious channel swims.

The South End Rowing Club conducts short swims from the Golden Gate or Pier 39 to the clubhouse and nearby locations. They also organize medium-length swims that include cross-current swims from Alcatraz, double Alcatrazes over to Alcatraz and back—called Bump and Runs, or Round Trip Alcatrazes—swims from Angel Island, Bridge to Bridge swims, or Sausalito to the club swims. Their longer swims include Point Bonita to the club; Candlestick Park to the club; and Bay Bridge to Ocean Beach, which they call "Bay 2 Breakers." Each is about ten miles long. Angel Island, round-trip, takes about two and a half hours to complete.

The South End Rowing Club also hosts a famous race

called the Alcatraz Invitational—a 1.25-mile open water swim from a point abeam to Alcatraz Island and back to the South End Rowing Clubhouse, at the foot of the Hyde Street Pier in San Francisco. They often host six hundred swimmers. It is a fun swim. Swimmers are shuttled out in groups on a ferryboat to Alcatraz Island. The swimmers jump into the water one at a time and swim across an area near where the bay flows into the Pacific. There's nothing quite as beautiful as the Golden Gate Bridge illuminated in the bright morning sunlight, spanning the bay from Mount Mason to the Marin Headlands. You see the yachts in Yacht Harbor, and in front of you the opening in the seawall—the entrance to the South End and Dolphin Clubhouse—Ghirardelli Square, the elegant tall ships in the National Park, and off to your left, all of Fisherman's Wharf, Coit Tower, and the deep blue bay waters that flow past the famous piers beyond Bay Bridge ten miles in the distance. The energy level for the Alcatraz Invitational is always extremely high. Often the club allows other groups to join, or supports a special cause.

One year, Bill Wygant was asked by Jeff Pokonosky, a swimmer in the Encinitas area, if Jake, his golden retriever, could swim in the Alcatraz race. Bill discussed it with the club, and they thought it was a great idea; then Bill called me, and I thought so, too, but I asked him many of the same questions I'd ask a human swimmer: How much has Jake trained for Alcatraz? If he's used to swimming off San Diego, will he have time to acclimate to the cooler water temperatures in the San Francisco Bay? He could go into hypothermia, just like a human swimmer. Will they have a support boat for Jake and be able to pull him out if he aspirates water? Will they have a vet on call? Has Jake swum in choppy water and in water with strong currents? Will he be distracted, swimming with a large group of people? Will he stay with Jeff? Is there a way to keep him away from the other swimmers, since he might bump into other swimmers and unintentionally scratch them? While most swimmers love dogs, not all swimmers do, and having a dog on board may stress them out. Can Jeff keep Jake on a leash before the swim, and set off with the lead group, and swim to a designated rowboat?

Bill discussed these questions with Jeff, who said that the dog had had a health check and was in great shape. Jake was swimming up to two miles a day in the waters off Encinitas and running on the beach and retrieving tennis balls. He was used to going in and out of the surf, and he sometimes swam in the afternoon in choppy water. He would get to San Francisco a few days early to acclimate to the cooler water temperature.

On the day of the Alcatraz race, swimmers set off in manageable groups, with the fastest swimmers in the first group, the second-fastest swimmers in the next group, and slower groups after that. Jake set off with Jeff amid the fastest swimmers, and they swam about one hundred yards off to the left of the other swimmers. Jake saw the pack of swimmers take off, and he wanted to race with the pace and beat the lead swimmer. Jeff knew that the pace was too fast for Jake and persuaded him to slow down. But when Jake saw the other swimmers passing him, he started picking up his pace again. Jeff had to keep holding him back so he would be able to complete the swim.

Jake's coat kept him warm, but Jeff was cold at the end of their swim. They were greeted by cheering crowds, and once they caught their breath, they stayed on the beach to cheer on the incoming swimmers. The swimmers cheered one another on, and family and friends wrapped them up in warm towels, jackets, and blankets as they emerged from the water and handed them hot drinks. It was a great day. That is what is so special about open water swimming: Everyone supports one another.

Other West Coast Swim Coaches and Groups

La Jolla Cove, near San Diego, is another great place to train. Swimmers of all ages and abilities swim in the La Jolla Cove. Bob West has swum there for years. He is a kingpin there—he knows every swimmer and every visiting swimmer and is always prepared to introduce and pair up swimmers based on their speed and compatibility. Once a high school football coach, and for years an open water swimmer, Bob encourages swimmers, educates them, and makes sure they have a chance to learn from other swimmers, including some who have swum the English Channel and San Pedro Channel.

East Coast Swim Coaches and Groups

The Coney Island Brighton Beach Open Water Swimmers (CIBBOWS) are well known for their open water swims off Brighton Beach and elsewhere in the New York City area. They are an established group with a core of very competent members who welcome new swimmers. It is great to have other people to swim with, to pace with, and to share the swimming experience with. They are knowledgeable about open water training, and some members of the group have swum across the English Channel and San Pedro Channel (see Sources for website address; page 299).

A great open water training group in East Hampton, New York, is YMCA Open Water Swim Training (YOWST), through the YMCA East Hampton RECenter and coached by Tim Treadwell. Tim is a beach lifeguard, marine safety officer, open water swimmer, and coach of a masters program that travels to Bermuda for a winter open water swim. See Sources (page 299) for his contact information.

There are three open water swims in East Hampton sponsored by East Hampton Volunteer Ocean Rescue (see Sources for the website with event details; page 299).

The Sea Monkeys in Seal Beach, California, train along

the shore of Seal Beach for most of the year and have a history of lifeguard participation in the workouts.

Santa Barbara Swimming Association conducts open water swims and channel swims and have experience supporting some technical and challenging swims (see Sources for website address; page 300).

Other U.S. Swim Coaches and Groups

Waikiki Swim Club is Hawaii's oldest club devoted to open water swimming (see Sources for website address; page 300).

Vision Quest Coaching in the Lake Michigan area works with experienced channel swimmers (see Sources for website address; page 300).

Masters long-distance world record holder and former University of Texas swimming coach Dr. Keith Bell, along with Sandy Neilson-Bell, my college swim team buddy and Olympic triple gold medalist, have created numerous open water swimming events in the Austin, Texas, area, including an open water stage race: the Tex Robertson Highland Lakes Challenge (see Sources for website address; page 300). This race takes place over a five-day period in five of the upper highland lakes in Texas hill country. They also host the October Lake Travis Relay (see Sources for website address; page 300), an approximately twelve-mile relay just outside Austin. It provides a challenge for six-man relay team members, as well as a limited number of solo swimmers. You can join the American Swimming Association's mailing list for an updated calendar of these and other open water races at their website (see Sources for website address; page 300).

International Swim Coaches and Groups

There are also overseas open water swimming groups and associations. They have members who are experienced open water swimmers.

Australia Surf Lifesaving Association: www.sls.com.au
England: www.brightonsc.co.uk
British Long Distance Swimming Association:
    www.bldsa.org.uk
Jersey Long Distance Swimming Club:
    www.jerseyseaswims.org
Serpentine Swimming Club:
    serpentineswimmingclub.com
The ASS Southeastern Region:
    www.southeastswimming.org
South Africa has an active open water swimming commu-
    nity, especially in Cape Town: www.capeswim.com

Another way to find an open water swimming coach is to attend some open water swimming competitions. You will meet other open water swimmers, see their coaches, and be able to observe how the coaches interact with their swimmers. If you are coming to the competition from out of your area, you can ask coaches at the event if they know coaches in your area. There is a strong network within the swimming community, and most coaches will try to help you.

Triathlon Coaches and Groups

John Martin, with communications and media relations for USA Triathlon, recommended taking a look at USA Triathlon's club listing page on their website to locate a nearby club. They also have a searchable database of coaches that can help you find a triathlon coach. See Sources (page 300) for the website addresses.

USA Triathlon is a great place to find out where triathlons will occur throughout the year and network with other triathletes and open water swimmers.

Lani Ralston is a friend who competes in triathlons, Ironman, ultra-marathon runs, and open water swims. She trains and swims on the East Coast and said that the open water swimming areas are well-kept secrets. She explained that if you just jump in the ocean or a lake where a lifeguard is not on duty, you will get a rather hefty fine, and the coast guard levies some penalties, too. Local triathlon clubs usually have information on which boat launch areas are okay with open water swimming, offer group swim times, and can guide athletes to open water swim coaches. Usually, you have to be a member to access forums and get this information. Sometimes a race's website will have this kind of information on a training page.

Lani said that a number of organizations put on triathlons. Ironman is a brand name owned by the World Triathlon Corporation (WTC). There are lots of races with a similar 2.4-mile (3.8-kilometer) swim, 112-mile (180.2-kilometer) bike ride, and 26.2-mile (45.1-kilometer) run. They typically are called Iron Distance races to avoid legal problems and are often run by other companies, such as Revolution3 (Rev3), or local clubs. USA Triathlon is the governing body of the sport, just like USA Swimming or Track and Field. You have to buy a license from them to participate in a tri.

Rev3 is different from the Ironman-branded races. Rev3 (see Sources for website address; page 300) is oriented toward customer service and families. They usually start and finish their races at amusement parks, where families get in for free and can enjoy themselves while the athletes are out racing. This series started in Connecticut, and in the past I have met both the female and male Ironman world champions there, as well as raced with them. All of these organizations are resources for finding a qualified open water swimming coach and finding friends to train with.

Chapter 4

Technical Skills for Open Water Swimming

Swimming through the open water can be very Zenlike. For many athletes, it is a time when they meditate. The world is reduced to their swimming and the sea. They hear the rhythm of their strokes, the crack and splash of the water as their hands enter the sea. They hear the sounds of their inhale and exhale and the bubbles bouncing out of their mouths. They watch the bubbles stream off their fingertips. They hear the sounds of their feet popping out of the water and the rhythm of the splashes. They hear the sounds of the waves crashing on shore, the burst of energy released into the ocean when a bird breaks the water and captures a fish. They hear the sound of the wind as it moves across the water, and the trill of the windblown waves.

SWIMMING SKILLS REQUIRED

Swimming in open water feels different from swimming in a swimming pool. The salt water makes you float higher, and the fresh water feels good against your skin. Whether you are swimming in salt or fresh or pool water, you don't swim *on* the water, you swim *through* the water.

One of biggest mistakes swimmers make is trying to swim on top of the water and fighting the water to stay up. They tend to shorten their swimming stroke, lift their heads, and drop their hips so that they are more vertical. This makes swimming difficult and causes some people to feel like they are sinking, which isn't true. Everyone floats, and everyone floats at a different level in the water according to body type, percent body fat and how well it is distributed, lung volume—how much air is brought into the lungs and residual volume—and how much air remains in the lungs after exhalation.

Your lungs are like two balloons in your back, and when you are relaxed, they fill with air and make you more buoyant. When you aren't relaxed in the water, the breaths that you take are usually shorter, and the lungs do not fill as much. The more relaxed you are in the water, the easier it is to breathe, the more your lungs fill with air, and the more you will float.

BREATHING DRILLS

A lot of swimmers don't exhale in a relaxed way and don't get all the air out on an exhale to make room for the new air coming in, so their breathing is tight and they are often breathless. They just can't seem to get enough air. This throws off their stroke, and they can't relax in the water. Bobbing helps you regulate your breathing. Bobbing drills are done in the shallow end of the swimming pool or in a placid, stingray-free bay or other area of calm water. They are fun, and they help you feel the lift—buoyancy—when you are in the water.

~ Go into water that is waist- to shoulder-deep.
~ Stand up, take a breath, and drop down under the water till your knees are bent.

~ Push off the bottom and exhale slowly.

~ Watch the bubbles roll out of your nose and mouth.

~ Do ten to fifteen bobs really slowly and let yourself relax.

~ When this drill begins to feel automatic, do ten more bobs. Have fun. Play with them. Blast off the bottom and drop under the water. Exhale slowly.

~ If you are getting water up your nose, it is because you aren't exhaling through your nose. Practice ten bobs with your mouth closed and blow out through your nose during each bob.

~ When this feels automatic, do ten to fifteen bobs slowly and breathe out through your mouth and nose.

Swimmers in the open water who breathe on only one side are blind on one side and compensate by lifting their heads to see what's going on around them. Every time they lift their heads, their hips drop in the water, which immediately increases resistance and inhibits speed, so they have to increase their energy output to compensate for the increased resistance. In order to swim efficiently, you need to bilateral-breathe. It is important that swimmers lift their heads to navigate, establish their position in the water, and check for boaters and surfers, but that can become a bad habit and a way of compensating for not breathing on both sides.

Bilateral breathing enables you to adjust to the environment. If you are swimming in windy conditions and you are breathing only on one side, there is a good chance you will breathe in water. Not a good thing. Choking on water is uncomfortable, distracting, and ultimately may affect the outcome of a swim by making you sick. If you are able to breathe on both sides of your body, you open up more options.

Years ago, on my swim across Cook Strait between the North and South islands of New Zealand, the wind was blowing constantly at forty-five knots. The visibility on my windward side was reduced to zero. Waves were slamming into my face and I couldn't get a breath; I just kept breathing water. Suddenly, it occurred to me that I could breathe only on the right side and not drink water. My stroke was no longer balanced, but at least I could keep swimming, and when the wind shifted, I was able to go back to breathing on both sides of my body.

Some swimmers, especially those who have been swimming for many years, think that it is difficult to breathe on both sides of their bodies and resist doing so, but this drill makes learning how to bilateral-breathe easy. When they start breathing on both sides, they immediately feel how much better it is to swim this way.

Bilateral Breathing Drill

Method:

~ Lie on your right side, as if you are going to swim side-stroke, with your right arm extended above your head and the other arm resting on your side.
~ Put your face in the water and blow bubbles. Take a breath when needed.
~ Kick six to eight times on your side.
~ Take a stroke with your left arm and use the core of your body to roll all the way over to the other side of your body. Make sure you are using your core to roll over. You will get a lot of power and strength from your core.
~ With your left arm extended, let your right arm rest on your side as you kick on your side six to eight times with your face in the water.
~ You want to maintain a straight line in the water. Usually, swimmers are more balanced on one side than the other. Sometimes it takes a little more concentration and work on balance to kick on one side as opposed to the other. But this exercise will help you balance your stroke

and also swim in a straighter line. It is easy to see which swimmers in the open water have a balanced stroke. Those who are not balanced will swim in the direction of their dominant side, off to the right or the left, and not maintain a straight line.

~ This drill will also help you maintain a horizontal position and enable you to move efficiently through the water. You will be rotating from one side of your body to the other and reinforcing that your arm stroke is done in conjunction with the rotation of your body, so that you are pulling with your core as well as your arms. If you do not use your core with your arm strokes, you will not swim efficiently. You will be swimming flat on the water, and if you are using only your arms, the muscles in your arms will fatigue more rapidly and you will tire sooner.

~ This drill will also help you develop a stronger core and arms and legs, which will help you increase your power, speed, and endurance when you are swimming.

Breathing and Breath-Holding Drill

In the swimming pool, when you turn your head to breathe, you can count on getting a full breath of air; in the open water, if the water is choppy, there are no guarantees. It's no fun breathing water. Not only is it uncomfortable when your mouth is full of water, but it causes you to abruptly stop swimming, and that throws you completely off your pace.

One of the drills you can do to prepare for choppy water is to practice turning your head to breathe without taking a breath.

~ Swim freestyle two hundred strokes and breathe every three strokes to warm up.

~ Swim freestyle one hundred more strokes at your pace, and breathe every third stroke. Every once in a while, turn your head to breathe on the third stroke without actually taking a breath. Take a breath on your fourth stroke.

~ Make sure that you are doing this drill with a buddy, so he or she can check on you to make sure you're okay and check for boat traffic. If you suddenly find you really need to breathe on the third stroke, take a breath. The point of this drill is to learn how to avoid breathing in water.

~ Swim one hundred more strokes and repeat this drill.

~ Once you feel comfortable changing your breathing pattern, swim in mildly choppy water. As you gain more experience and confidence, you will be able to feel the waves around your head and judge the times when you can take a breath and when you'll have to wait and turn to the opposite side to breathe.

~ For intermediate and advanced swimmers: There are times when the wind and waves are so large that it's impossible to breathe on one side of your body. Breathe on the side you can get air, and have someone in a kayak or boat, or on a paddleboard beside you, guide you and be there for safety.

HEAD POSITION IN THE WATER

One of the most important considerations in open water swimming is your head position. Remember Newton's third law of motion: For every action, there is an equal and opposite reaction. *Everything* moves relative to *everything* else. If you lift your head while you're swimming, your hips will drop in the water. You will immediately feel the increased resistance of the water against your body. Your legs and hips will be like an anchor dragging through the water. Swimming in this way requires a lot more energy, and you will tire faster than if you keep your hips on the water's surface.

Often I think of it like this: Your head leads the way, and your body follows.

There are two situations when people lift their heads. The first is when they breathe, and the second is when they navigate. The way to swim more efficiently is to make sure you are rotating your head when you breathe; don't lift your head. If you do the bilateral breathing drill, you will feel the roll of your body and sense the right time to breathe. It will be easy to turn your head to breathe. If you are swimming flat on the water and you aren't rotating to breathe, you will tend to lift your head. This is a bad habit. Depending on the distance that you are swimming, lifting your head may decrease your speed by minutes or even hours, because your reduced speed may cause you to miss a tide.

It is good to lift your head to navigate and to check for boats or vessels around you. Toward the end of a swim, I have developed a bad habit of lifting my head to see how much farther I have to swim to shore. The way I've tried to break that habit is by counting up to a thousand strokes, then giving myself permission to lift my head and see if I've made progress.

Some swimmers tend to bury their heads in the water. If you bury your head, your hips will float higher on the water, but you will also create more water resistance against your head, which will slow you down.

The solution for the most efficient head position is to let your head float and find its ideal position in the water. Relax your neck muscles. Imagine the water is a pillow supporting your head.

Another way to find your head position is by doing a drill in which you exaggerate your head's movement. Swim two hundred strokes with your head out of the water, then swim two hundred strokes with your head buried in the water. Repeat this drill five times so you swim a total of one thousand strokes. You will feel how much more energy it takes to swim with your head out of the water, like a water polo player, and you will feel how much extra energy you use to press your face into the water. Now place your head in the water halfway between the lifted and the buried head position and let your head float. You will immediately feel yourself moving through the water, and you will feel how much easier it is to swim. You will increase your efficiency, speed, and endurance.

FEELING THE WATER TO SWIM FASTER

Years ago, Don Gambril told our swim team to go to a pet store and watch the fish swim. He told us to notice how the fish used tiny sculling motions with their fins and explained that the best swimmers in the world use these sculling motions when they swim.

We watched goldfish swim across the fish tank. Using tiny sculling motions, they flew across the tank. Don Gambril asked us to imagine that we were swimming like the goldfish. Swimmers often imagine things because they spend so much time in their heads while they're swimming, but this time it would improve our stroke mechanics.

George Block and Laura Cox, at Alamo Area Aquatic Association in Texas, developed a series of sculling drills that will help you feel the water and "find new water." Finding new water is one of the most important concepts of swimming. The more efficiently swimmers can find new water, the faster they will propel themselves through the water.

Sculling

Whether you are a beginning, intermediate, or advanced swimmer, these sculling drills are essential to swimming. They are the basis of your stroke. A musician practices scales to find the right fingering on an instrument, to create the perfect sound and tempo. Similarly, you need to practice these skills to refine your swimming technique and find your perfect pitch through the water.

Sculling drills will help you find new water and will help you find the correct placement of your hands in the water. They will help you improve all of your strokes, though the focus of the drills described below is on freestyle, since the majority of open water swimmers use freestyle during their swims.

If you do each drill in sequence, as described below, your arms will naturally go to the right positions when you are pulling, and you will find the ultimate arm stroke unique to your own body. The drills will also make sure you "pop" your elbow up during the pull phase of your arm stroke during freestyle. This will enable you to maintain a high elbow on your underwater pull, keep pressure on the water, and pull more water so that you can swim more efficiently and faster.

Superman Scull and Drill

This drill helps you get a handle on the water, and it works on the catch part of your stroke.

~ Float facedown on the water and extend your hands out in front of your head as if you are Superman flying through the water. Scull with your arms extended straight out above your head.

~ Keep your hands relaxed and fingers together but also relaxed. Press slightly down on the water and pitch (or angle) your palms forward to move the water toward your feet by moving your hands side to side. Do not slice the water; do not push the water with your palms facing each other; and do not move your hands straight back (or pull) toward your feet. Feel the water move. The way you scull may be slightly different than your swimming buddy's because your body type, flexibility, and strength may be different. Some swimmers say they create a J shape and an inverted J shape with their fingertips, and some swimmers say they create a small U shape with their fingertips when they are sculling. You may make other motions, depending on your body type and strength level. The most important thing is to maintain constant pressure on the water with your hands. You will also feel the pressure of the water against your forearms.

~ For a beginning swimmer, scull two hundred times easy. Concentrate on feeling the way you are moving your hands. Feel the water against your fingers and palms. Notice how quickly your tiny hand movements propel you through the water.

~ Make sure your neck and shoulders are relaxed. If you tighten your body during this drill, you will be wasting energy. Focus on your energy on your sculling.

~ Make sure you roll your head to breathe. Breathe on both sides, and notice where you are in the water. If you are doing this drill with your swimming buddy nearby, close your eyes and feel your hands moving the water. (By closing your eyes, you eliminate all distractions.) You'll find that this drill is relaxing and fun.

~ If you are an intermediate open water swimmer, continue this drill by sculling two hundred times at a moderate speed. Make sure you are holding on to the water, even when you are increasing your speed.

~ Repeat the drill by sculling one hundred times again at a slow pace, then swim four hundred strokes freestyle at a slow pace. Feel the sculling motion when you catch the water at the start of your arm stroke. Swim freestyle four hundred more strokes at a moderate pace. Make sure you catch the water and keep constant pressure on it. You will feel the catch part of your pull (when your hand first enters the water) immediately become stronger.

~ Swim relaxed freestyle for two hundred more strokes and move on to the Superman drill.

~ If you are an intermediate or advanced open water swimmer, continue to alternate between two hundred sculls slow and two hundred sculls moderate for a mile, depending on the distance you're swimming that day. If you are swimming cold or in cold water, you will notice that your heat production will be a lot lower than when you are swimming freestyle. If the water is cool or cold, after eight hundred sculls, swim eight hundred strokes freestyle to increase your heat production. If you are warm, continue the sculling drills for the mile, but if you have cooled down, do not continue sculling; swim freestyle. Make sure you and your swimming buddy are monitoring each other. Keep your eyes open when your buddy has his/her eyes shut.

~ Swim freestyle for a mile, concentrating on the catch of your stroke. You will feel how important it is to begin the sculling motion as soon as your hand enters the water. By doing the next drill, you will feel how your stroke progresses.

Windshield Wiper Scull and Drill

~ If you are working out in the open water, imagine that you are lying on your stomach on the side of the pool with your head and arms extended over the edge and your hands in the water. Imagine that you are keeping your elbows just above the waterline. Move your hands in and out with your palms pitched backward like windshield wipers.

~ Float in the water on your stomach, with your face in the water, in the windshield wiper position. Open your armpits and move your hands in and out with your palms pitched backward and fingertips pointed toward the bottom. Some think of their arms moving like pendulums. Make sure you are moving your arms side to side, not back and forth.

~ If you are a beginning swimmer, do the windshield wiper drill for two hundred strokes. Make sure your fingers touch under the centerline of your body, and then sweep them out until your arms are extended. Notice how your hands are positioned under your chest. Feel the water pressure on your hands and forearms. Make sure to keep constant pressure on the water. If you slip water, you lose the power phase of your stroke.

~ Use the Superman drill for two hundred sculls at a slow rate, then two hundred sculls at a moderate rate. Remember when you speed up your hand movement that you need to keep holding on to the water. Relax your body and let your hands and arms work. Breathe when you need to breathe. Repeat this drill two more times.

~ To feel the sculling motion within your stoke, swim three hundred strokes freestyle, feeling the middle part of your arm stroke and the windshield wiper part of your stroke. You will notice an enormous difference. You will be able to feel how your hands are holding water and pressing it backward. You will feel much more power in your stroke.

~ If you are an intermediate or advanced swimmer, continue the Superman drill for a mile. Continue sculling, and increase your rate to four hundred sculls. Alternate between four hundred slow and four hundred moderate for a mile, then swim half a mile or up to a mile freestyle. Feel the windshield wiper's sculling motion within your arm's stroke. By focusing on this sculling motion, you will hold on to more water through the range of your stroke and swim faster.

~ Continue your workout. Swim one mile freestyle. Think about the catch part of your stroke—the Superman scull and the under-your-body part of the stroke—in the windshield wiper scull and feel how you are integrating your stroke.

If you are sculling correctly, you will notice that your stroke rate—the number of strokes you take per minute—is slower. That's a good thing. It means that you are getting a hold on the water and pulling new water. You may also feel the added resistance of each arm stroke, which will make you stronger. As you work on this drill, you will gain a better feel for the water, and as you become stronger, you will be able to pull with more power and propel yourself faster.

Double-Dog Scull and Drill

This drill helps you work on the elbow pop of your stroke, which is essential in swimming freestyle. It helps you maintain a high elbow during your underwater pull. This is critical for maintaining pressure on the water. If you drop your elbow during the underwater pull, you'll slip water and lose the main power portion of your stroke.

~ Start with the outsweep of the Superman scull and then insweep with a windshield wiper scull and complete the double dog with an outsweep in the finish scull position with your hands snapping past your hips. Make sure your fingertips are pointed toward the ocean or lake bottom during the windshield wiper insweep and that your armpits stay open with your hands below your belly button.

~ For the beginning swimmer, scull one hundred times slowly and lift your head to breathe when you need to; then scull one hundred times at a moderate rate. Focus on your hand and chest movements. Feel the lift of the water as you bring your hands toward each other during the sculling phase, and feel your chest drop into the water as you move your hands out toward your sides. Repeat this drill four times, then swim freestyle for four hundred strokes and feel the double-dog phase of the scull in your freestyle.

~ If you are an intermediate or advanced swimmer, continue the drill for a mile. Alternate between sculling slowly and sculling at a moderate speed. Even though this drill is repetitious, it is important to stay focused. Do not daydream. Pay attention to how your hands are moving. Feel the strength of your hands and the powerful water movement you create when you are sculling.

~ Integrate this drill by swimming one mile freestyle, and concentrate on the downward-dog scull within your freestyle stroke.

Finish Scull and Drill

The finish scull helps you work on the finish part of your arm stroke.

~ Lie on your stomach with your face in the water. Place your hands under your hips with your arms held in by your sides and your fingertips pointed down toward the bottom of the lake or ocean.

~ Move your hands in a sculling motion in front of your hips. Concentrate on feeling the water. This is a part of the stroke where some swimmers slip water and lose a lot of power. Focus on strong movements. Breathe when you need to, by either lifting your head or rolling to the side.

~ If you are a beginning swimmer, do three hundred finish sculls at a slow speed to warm up. Do three hundred sculls at a moderate speed, then three hundred sculls at a slow speed. Take your time and feel your hands move the water. Do three hundred sculls at a moderate speed. Maintain your hold on the water.

~ Swim six hundred strokes freestyle and feel the sculling motion that you use during the finish part of your stroke.

~ If you are an intermediate or advanced swimmer, continue this drill for a mile. Increase your sculling rate to four hundred sculls at a slow pace. Alternate between that and four hundred sculls at a moderate pace.

~ Swim one mile freestyle and concentrate on the finish part within your arm stoke.

Integration of Sculling Drills

When you are swimming freestyle and you integrate these sculling drills, your hands will move from one sculling position to the next, automatically creating the perfect S curve under your body that coaches and swimmers talk about. You will discover your stroke—a stroke that is unique to you and perfect for your body.

As you become more in tune with your body and more comfortable in the water in your own stroke, you will want to change around the sculling drills to create variety in your workout. You may vary the distance and the speed that you scull. As your sculling becomes second nature, increase your speed and scull fast. Mix it up. Do the drills in different orders and combinations. Do all the scull drills first and then swim. The more variety you can create within your workout, the more interesting it will be, and the more likely you are to enjoy your swim and have fun.

Increasing Your Feel of the Water and Drill

Sometimes when you remove stimulation and focus on one sense—for example, closing your eyes and listening to your environment—you are able to heighten your awareness of what's occurring around you. It's the same with swimming. By reducing the size of your hand, this drill will give you more of a feel for the water and, in turn, a stronger pull.

~ When you are swimming, ball up your fingers into fists and swim with your hands fisted for one hundred meters. You will immediately notice that you have reduced the size of your "paddle" and that you are not holding on to water. You will also feel the resistance of the water more against your forearm.

~ Now swim one hundred meters with your hand open like a paddle, the way you normally swim. You'll feel the path that your hand makes through the water. The resistance should be constant. You will be able to feel when you are holding on to the water and getting successful pulls and when you are slipping water and not getting successful pulls.

~ Alternate one-hundred-meter swims with your hand shaped like a ball, and then relaxed like a paddle, during the warm-up portion of your workout. This drill is like a tuning fork for your swimming stroke; it helps you to focus on the biomechanics of your swimming stroke and your efficiency. While most open water swimmers use freestyle as their main swimming stroke, you can also use this drill for butterfly, backstroke, and breaststroke.

It is important to use different strokes during your workouts, especially if you are swimming long distances. This serves several purposes: It will give you a variety of swimming skills to work out; it will keep your mind active; and it will enable you to work and stretch different muscle groups so that you can build overall body strength.

If you swim primarily freestyle, and you roll over on your back and swim backstroke, you will stretch out the muscles you use for swimming freestyle and at the same time strengthen the muscles you use for backstroke.

When you swim breaststroke and butterfly, you focus on the catch part of your stroke (the front part of the stroke when your hands enter and start pulling the water). By working on this part of the stroke while doing breaststroke and butterfly, you will gain a better catch when you are swimming freestyle. This, in turn, will help you swim faster but also enjoy being in the open water more.

When you swim backstroke, it is more difficult to sight buoys and piers to swim on course, so you have to be even more alert to your surroundings. Use a reference point beyond your feet and line up with that point in order to stay on course. Also, swim inside a buoy line and with another competent swimmer, or have a kayaker or paddler beside you. Glance toward shore to make sure you're swimming in a straight line; if the lifeguard stations or the people or buildings on land look closer and then farther away, you are weaving in and out and need to pull more evenly with your arms. Feel the water movement and figure out if you are in a current that is moving you off course, then compensate by turning into or out of the current.

Swimming backstroke will help you hone your open water skills, but just as important, you will gain a different perspective and see the beauty around you. You can see the depths and color changes in the sky; you can watch the clouds sail across the sky and how they merge and slip apart and change in shape and texture and color. You can watch seabirds—gulls, terns, pelicans, ducks, grebes, cormorants, phoebes, geese, great blue herons, sandpipers, willets, sanderlings, swans, and many other water birds—circling, diving, flapping, and gliding. You can watch the movement of the sun, the way it illuminates the water, and the way its rays are altered by the clouds. You can see sailboats, kite surfers, and windsurfers in the distance, and tell the direction of the wind, and know where the current will grow stronger or where it will diminish. You can watch airplanes and helicopters move across the constantly changing sky, and enjoy seeing the movement of life around you.

When you swim butterfly, you focus on the dolphin motion of your body. You work on developing the power of your core and your dolphin kick. You work on the strength of your arms and the rhythm of the stroke and breath. This helps you with your overall body conditioning. Your breathing pattern allows you to lift up for a breath and see what is directly in front of you, and when you drop underwater during the recovery, you can see what is below you.

You are focused on the worlds in front of and below you, and you're able to observe life beneath you, the kelp beds or coral reefs teeming with fish and crustaceans.

When you swim breaststroke, you can glide along the surface of the water, and as with butterfly, you transit two worlds, the place you are reaching toward and the world you are moving over. When you swim breaststroke, you can drive your arms forward and propel your stroke with a strong frog kick, but you can also use breaststroke as active recovery, in which you slow down, catch your breath, and take time to enjoy the feel of the water and the way your body moves through it.

Maintaining a Straight Line and Drill

One of the ways to swim in a straight line is to make sure you open your eyes when your face is in the water. If you are closing your eyes, you will be blind for a few moments, which will affect your balance, and you will veer off course.

A drill to help you maintain a straight line is to swim with your eyes closed. This drill must be done with a buddy swimming right beside you at all times in a safe swimming area. Your swimming buddy will be there to watch out for you, and you will do the same for your buddy.

~ Close your eyes and swim parallel to shore for one hundred strokes.

~ Open your eyes, turn around, and check your route. Did you swim straight or veer to the right or the left?

~ If you did not swim in a straight line, you may be pulling and crossing over the midline under your body with one of your arms. The way to feel the midline of your body is to take your index finger, place it on your forehead, and run it down your face and body to create an imaginary line that cuts your body in half. If you veer to the left when you're swimming, you may be crossing the midline of your body with your right hand. If you veer to the right, you may be crossing under the midline of your body with your left hand.

~ You may be going off course because you're pulling stronger with one arm than the other.

~ Try the drill again. If you were crossing your midline with one hand, take a wider stroke so that you don't cross the midline. If you were pulling stronger with one arm than the other, concentrate on pulling the water with equal force.

All of these drills will help you balance in the water, keep you on a straighter course, and help you swim faster in the open water.

Chapter 5

Research

SELECTING A TRAINING AREA

While this section is mainly for beginning open water swimmers, every open water swimmer should take these steps before entering any waterway.

When you start open water swimming, you want to find a waterway that is relatively safe, where the water is clean, and where you can swim along the shoreline. Before you even enter the water, talk to the local experts who know the conditions. Go to lifeguard headquarters and talk with the older, experienced lifeguards who have spent years patrolling the beach and the waters. Those lifeguards will know great details about their beaches, and they will probably have many interesting stories that will tell you what to be aware of when you shuffle into the water.

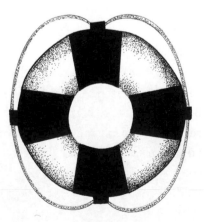

To get a complete idea of what the water is like, also talk with the local harbormaster, the coast guard, surfers, sailors, divers, fishermen, harbor patrol, and other experienced open water swimmers. If you begin in a lake, river, or stream that is within the bounds of a state or national park, such as Yellowstone Lake, the park rangers can provide a wealth of information about the water conditions, as well as how to respect and be aware of the bears and buffalo that live around the lake.

SCOUTING/WALKING THE WORKOUT COURSE

The best swim courses are those that are parallel to the beach. For years, my swimming friends and I have swum parallel to shore along a buoy line that stretches the length of the beach or just outside the wave break. There is no real need to swim out into deep water, especially when most boaters, windsurfers, kite surfers, and Jet Skiers are not looking for swimmers far offshore.

Walk along the beach and observe the training area. You will be able to see various landmarks, and when you enter the water, you'll recognize them and use them for navigation and to indicate the distance you have swum.

TIDAL CHARTS

Before any long-distance swim, you want to check the tides. Even when you're doing training swims, check on the tides. The swimmers at the South End Rowing Club in San Francisco always check the tides before they swim, because if they don't time the tide and their swim correctly, they can't make it back to the club. Tides will affect your workout times. If you swim back and forth along the coast, you will have the tide with you and against you, and you'll be able to see if you're on your pace, but if you're swimming only in one direction, it's hard to tell how fast you are going and whether you're fighting the tide or getting a push.

L. Tadeus said that the SEALs use tide tables to figure out training swims:

> You can find tide tables online easily. They are based on observations at specific locations—choose the one closest to your swim. A local marina near the swim location would have the most accurate charts. Occasionally, you get lucky and a particular section of a body of water has been thoroughly studied for some tangential purpose for which tides were necessary. Tidal predictions for these areas tend to be hyperaccurate but require creative research techniques to locate.

Tidal charts are very specific. The tides in the English Channel are different, for example, from the Irish Sea. Tidal charts are good only one year, because the tides change annually.

WATER TEMPERATURE

Always check the water temperature before you swim; it will give you an indication of how long you can swim that day. You'll also need to be aware of how you are feeling in the water, if you're too cold or too hot.

It is a good idea to have a journal to record the water temperature and your swim time and distance and how you felt during your workout, so you can see whether you're acclimating to the water temperature.

The water temperature is a good indicator of your estimated time in the water. When I first started training for the Strait of Magellan swim, the water temperature was forty-two degrees—eight degrees colder than the waters off Santa Barbara, California, where I did the majority of training for the swim. Eight degrees was a huge difference.

The water in the Strait of Magellan felt so much colder than the Pacific. The first day I could stand in waist-deep water for twenty minutes. The next day I talked myself into swimming for twenty minutes, and I gradually added more time for each workout as I acclimated to the cold. The water temperature indicated how frequently I would drink warm fluids.

Water temperature also played a major role in my Gulf of Aqaba swims. There the water temperature was eighty degrees, and the air temperature was ninety degrees Fahrenheit. By learning how hot the air and water were, I realized that I needed to slow down so I wouldn't go into hyperthermia (overheating during the swim), and I knew I had to drink cool fluids every twenty minutes. Just as I got acclimated to the cold waters off Chile, I had to acclimate to the hot water temperatures between Egypt, Israel, and Jordan.

WATER QUALITY

Many of us swim because it is fun and something that makes us healthy and happy. Swimming in the ocean adds a lot to our lives. But water quality fluctuates daily depending on the waterway, the time of year, and what might have been dumped in the waterway. We need to pay attention.

Nick Bolin, the Seal Beach, California, safety officer/lifeguard, offered the following comments and recommendations:

~ Water quality can be a concern when swimming in the ocean. Many counties regularly check the water quality. If water contamination is detected, lifeguards and coastal agencies are notified, and signs are posted on the beach advising swimmers and surfers not to enter the water. Always check with the lifeguards or county health departments about water quality before you enter the water. For example, the Orange County Health Care Agency states: "The Environmental Health staff advised swimmers that levels of bacteria can rise significantly in the ocean and bay waters adjacent to storm drains, creeks and rivers during and after rainstorms. The elevated levels of bacteria can continue for a period of at least 3 days depending upon the intensity of the rain and the volume of the runoff. Swimmers should avoid coastal waters impacted by discharging storm drains, creeks and rivers, and beach users should avoid contact with any runoff on the beach during dry or wet weather conditions."

~ Because water quality is dependent on so many factors and thus in constant flux, be sure to check with the state health department on water quality before you get into the water.

~ Don't swim during moderate to heavy rainstorms and especially near storm drains. A Navy SEAL said that they have experienced serious problems with water quality in such conditions. He said, "We had an entire dive team come down with skin lesions all over their bodies after a good rain in Pearl Harbor. At first, the Dive Medical Officers suspected cutus marmorata, a form of decompression illness. Turns out they had chemical burns from runoff contaminated by all the crystal meth labs in the mountains of Oahu. Beaches are always closing on the south shore of Oahu due to sewage spills."

All sorts of contaminants wash into the water when it's raining, as well as a lot of debris. I've run headfirst into floating logs and garbage. You may not want to miss your ocean workouts, but if you're swimming in polluted water, you can contract an infection from high levels of bacteria and be out of the water a lot longer than a few days. This happened to me after swimming in Santa Monica Bay one day after a heavy rain. A group of swimmers who worked out in the area all the time said that the water was fine. What I realized later was that they might have built up some immunity to the bacteria in the water. I had my first bad sinus infection, and I had to stay out of the water for two weeks.

FOOD AND HYDRATION

One of the questions that I'm asked most often is: What do open water swimmers eat and drink during their swims?

Years ago, in Egypt, Kevin Murphy, one of the most accomplished open swimmers of all time, took me under his wing. Kevin was one of the funniest, kindest, and zaniest swimmers I'd ever met. Once, in Cairo, we were late for our workouts. At that time Kevin was competing for the title of swimming the English Channel the most number of times. I remember asking him, "What do you eat during your long swims?" He said, "Rice pudding and warm black tea."

I asked him why.

"Because it goes down as easily as it comes back up."

This did not seem like a good idea to me, and since then he's found a better solution for his swims. In long-distance open water swimming, you need to be able to hold down what you're eating and drinking. You don't want to vomit food and lose electrolytes—your energy source—and become dehydrated, and possibly attract dangerous fish.

Through the years, I've tried all kinds of drinks and foods. Quaker Oats helped sponsor my Beagle Channel swim. Before I traveled to Argentina, the CEO of Quaker Oats invited me to their laboratory to meet with the biochemist who created new flavored drinks for Gatorade and Quaker Oats.

The head of the research division led the way down white corridors to a lab where two biochemists, wearing white lab coats and thick glasses, both around thirty years old, told me that they were interested in developing a higher-carbohydrate drink that could be used for endurance sports. They wanted me to test it. They had been working to add mango to their sports drinks, and when they asked if that appealed and it didn't, they offered to create a new flavor for me.

The Beagle Channel, between Argentina and Chile, was my next scheduled swim. It had never been attempted. The water was cold, in the low forties, and the sea was very rough, due to frequent storms. "Could they create a tropical drink that would make me think of swimming between tropical islands? Could you make a piña colada carbo-load drink?"

The head of the research division smiled. He said he had grown up in India, and he drank a lot of coconut milk, and that the flavor might be good for endurance sports, but you would probably want to use a light coconut flavor. The two scientists began discussing the biochemistry formulas for flavor. They spoke in numbers and codes because they had to keep their inventions secret. They turned to me and asked questions: "Do you want the drink to be sweet or only slightly sweet? Do you want it acidic, slightly acidic, or not acidic at all? Do you want more coconut flavor or more pineapple?" Each time they asked a question, they closed their eyes and pursed their lips as if sampling the drink they were creating in their minds.

The head of the research division also became excited about the idea of piña colada. He said he had grown up drinking pineapple juice, too, and he thought that the pineapple flavor was very nice but probably needed to be subtler than the coconut. The flavor scientists nodded in agreement, but they were looking intently at me, waiting for me to answer their questions.

The creamy flavor of the coconut might soothe my throat, and the not-too-sweet pineapple without acid would cut the salt residue in my mouth during the swim.

The only downside of the drink was that it sounded delicious cold, but I wasn't sure how it would taste warm. On a long swim in cold water, you need to be able to drink it warm in order to warm your core. How would hot pineapple taste?

Their brows furrowed as they considered how the flavor would be altered when they heated the drink. The head of the research division said, "Well, that is your new challenge," and they nodded and smiled and then asked me, "Do you want the drink in powder form or in liquid? Powder might be easier if you're traveling; you can just add it to water, and it's a lot lighter than carrying liquid."

A few months later, a large jar of powdered piña colada carbo-load arrived from their labs, and I tested it during my workouts. It tasted good when it was cool but not as good when it was hot. I was also concerned about drinking too much of the high-carbohydrate drink. I had not had a problem before, but friends who were marathon runners and cyclists told me that high-carbohydrate drinks could cause gas and diarrhea—not something you want to experience on any long-distance event. I made sure not to drink too much, and it gave me energy, although I like simple natural warm apple juice better, and I enjoy soft oatmeal raisin cookies because they float, and at times throughout a long swim, I want to eat something solid, not only drink fluids. I continued to search for foods and drinks that could be used on long swims, and discovered that my college roommates, who were Olympic swimmers, ate bowls of oatmeal before their big competitions. They said the oatmeal had staying power; they did not get hungry before their races, and it gave them energy.

Oatmeal works for me for the same reasons. But this quest to find what will work best before and during a long swim is something that continues to interest me. When I was on a speaking tour in Canada, I stayed a few nights at the Prince of Wales Hotel, and I tried their crème brûlée oatmeal. It was the best oatmeal I had ever eaten. I got up very early those two mornings so I had time to swim in the hotel pool, and during the workout, I looked forward to a steaming bowl of crème brûlée oatmeal, made with grainy steel-cut oats that had a nutty flavor, and plump apple slices, perfectly cooked, as if they had been stolen from an apple tart. The apples, perhaps Fuji or Pink Lady, were infused with cinnamon and nutmeg, mixed into the oatmeal, and covered with a fine layer of crème brûlée custard, then topped with a swizzle of real Canadian maple syrup. Some of it remained as golden syrup, and some of it was flamed momentarily until it was paper-thin crisp maple candy. While I worked out, I tried to figure out how this memorable breakfast feast could be made into an oatmeal cookie, but it might lend itself better to an oatmeal-apple muffin injected with a heart of crème brûlée.

As athletes, we always look for food/drinks that will be easy to eat and drink, that will digest easily, and most important, give us the sustained energy for endurance and the burst of energy we need for sprints, as well as be something we can look forward to during or even after a very long swim. It is interesting to note that in the last couple of years, a drink that a lot of people are using during endurance runs or triathlons is coconut water (serve it cool during warm swims), and the flavor researchers, chemists, and I created a variation on the coconut flavor more than thirty years ago.

Here are variables that affect food and drink choices:

~ If you're swimming in cold water, you will be looking for something warm to drink and eat to help warm your body and give you energy.

~ If you're swimming in warm water, you'll be looking for cool drinks and foods to help cool your body.

~ If you're swimming in cold salt water, you'll look for drinks that are not high in salt content, because you are already ingesting salt from the water.

~ If you're swimming in warm salt water, you will want to find a drink that tastes good, cools the body, and replaces electrolytes. If you're drinking a lot of salt water during rough warm-water swims, as I did in the Gulf of Aquaba, you might not want to add more salt to your system, and you may decide to drink fresh water and/or dilute the sports drink, as a lot of endurance athletes do. Whether you're in cold or hot water, make sure to get enough hydration.

~ When you are using warm fluids during a swim, make sure they aren't too hot, because your lips will be cooled to the temperature of the water, and if the fluid is hot, it will feel as if you are burning your lips.

~ In third-world countries, used bottles containing purified water are sometimes gathered up, filled with tap water, and resealed. If the tap water is full of bacteria that your system is not accustomed to, you can get sick. I've learned to purchase sparkling water (also called water with gas), because sparkling water cannot be put back in a reused bottle. Unscrew the bottle cap and let the gas out for a day or two before your swim or you'll be burping while you're swimming.

~ Salt water has a tendency to irritate the throat and make your tongue swell. If you are drinking and eating something with an acid base, it will irritate your throat.

~ For most swimmers in salt water, drinks with a milk base, cheese, and chocolate do not digest well.

~ High-carbohydrate drinks can cause gas, cramps, or gastric dumping (diarrhea).

Recently, I had breakfast with friends who are ultra-marathon runners and asked them what they ate before their races and during their hundred-mile runs. Often they eat peanut butter and jelly sandwiches, something that open water swimmers also eat, though we cut the sandwich into small pieces so they can be eaten easily while treading water.

The ultramarathon runners also eat half an avocado on runs. The avocado contains good fats that are not only healthy but also provide a long-term energy supply. Given that a lot of open water swimmers are swimming in salty environments, the avocado is something that is easy to eat, soothes the throat, and tastes good with the salt in your mouth.

It is important to stay hydrated during your workouts and your long-distance swims. The amount you hydrate depends on your own body's needs as well as water temperature and air temperature. Even in colder temperatures, you need to make sure you're drinking enough liquids.

Some swimmers hydrate before and after they swim, and on longer swims, they have a paddler, kayaker, or boat support person carry their fluid and sometimes a small cooler to keep their food chilled. The support people hand or toss the water bottles and food to swimmers, who tread water, do an eggbeater kick, or float. They do not touch the support craft or support people during the feeding period. Under English Channel and Catalina Channel swimming rules, and during competitive open water swims, swimmers will be disqualified if they touch the support craft or support people. This is to ensure that they do not rest on the side of the boat or support craft and complete their swim under their own power.

When I swam the English Channel, I carried warm fluids in cleaned shampoo bottles that I used as water bottles. I stopped every hour or two to hydrate and feed. My father had advised me to feed every hour to maintain my blood sugar level and energy level, but I wanted to break the world record and did not want to waste time feeding, or stop and get cold. Years later, I realized that I made a mistake. It would have been wiser to feed and drink more frequently and have more energy to swim; I may have swum much faster.

Now most swimmers who are doing open water swims

of ten miles (16 kilometers) or more feed or drink every twenty to thirty minutes, and most of them use warm fluids, because the English Channel temperatures range from 56 to 66 degrees F (13.3 to 18.8 degrees C). Manufacturers such as L.L. Bean, Eddie Bauer, and Starbucks have created insulated water bottles that are much easier to use than shampoo bottles.

Some swimmers, such as Murph Renford, get seasick or don't hold down food very well. Murph has spent a lot of time working with a sports nutritionist to figure out what he needs to eat. He said, "I have a gel, followed by 250 milliliters (8.4 ounces) of water at the one-hour mark, then every thirty minutes thereafter for the duration of the swim." Murph uses Shotz Energy Gel—always mango passion, he tells me (see Sources for website address; page 300). "It is far from an exact science," he continues, "but it seems to works for me. Having said that, I hate feeding time, and I think a lot of this comes down to my seasickness and dizziness when I stop swimming."

Murph said that during his English Channel swim, he was feeding every forty-five minutes with 600 milliliters (20.2 ounces) of water, but that amount was hard to digest. For the Manhattan swim, he reduced the feeds to every forty minutes with 400 milliliters (13.5 ounces) of water, and even that was too much to digest. He added that a thirty-minute feed time with less water seemed to work best for him.

He said the sports nutritionist recommended that he drink approximately 1,200 milliliters (40.5 ounces) of water/fluid every sixty minutes, which equates to 600 milliliters (20.2 ounces) every thirty minutes, "and for me and, I believe, most swimmers, this is not physically possible. I have no doubt that she is right, but the practicality of achieving this as a swim progresses would be near impossible."

Everyone is different, and the most important thing regarding feeding is to figure out what works best for you.

There are swimmers who methodically test different foods and liquids and are all set for their swims, and then they travel overseas and meet swimmers who, with the best intentions, tell them that they've got it wrong, they need to drink or eat something else. It is a mistake to try something else a few days' before a swim. It may not sit well, and can cause an upset stomach and a bad swim.

L. Tadeus discussed food options with me. He said that when the trainees are in intense training, they eat thousands of calories per day, and even then, some of the trainees can't hold on to their body weight. The trainers work on educating the trainees about nutrition, and like athletes, each SEAL works on what will work best for him. When L. Tadeus was a SEAL trainee, he and his buddy were doing a five-mile swim. They were swimming the combat stroke, side by side, when his swim buddy suddenly unzipped his wet suit and pulled out a plastic bag with two slices of pizza inside and handed one to him. He said it was the best pizza he had ever eaten.

When asked about supplements, L. Tadeus cautioned, "I believe you should specifically mention avoiding creatine-filled supplements for endurance athletes. We have had a couple of trainees overheat and nearly die from using this in the program."

To find out why this occurred, I contacted Charlie Nagurka, MD, an internist. He wrote, "There is little reliable information available regarding creatine. Most of the information on the Web is from sellers of supplements. It can cause kidney damage" (see Sources for more information; page 300).

Chapter 6

Into the Open Water

Going from pool swimming to open water swimming is like going from a fish tank to the ocean. Remember how badly Nemo wanted to escape the tank? The swimming pool is a stable and controlled environment, and in the open water, anything can happen. That's what makes swimming in the open water challenging, interesting, fun, and exciting. But because the water is always in flux, open water swimmers need to be aware, alert, and always in tune with what is happening around them. Otherwise, they can put themselves in dangerous situations.

Walk the beach before you get into the water. Study the area where you will be swimming. Can you see where the water goes from a lighter color to a darker color? The darker blue indicates deeper water. This darker blue tells you where the beach drops off and where you have to begin your swim. If this is an ocean beach, the dark to light area often indicates where the waves will rise and begin to break. All of this is important when you're entering the water.

THE STINGRAY SHUFFLE

Stingrays are very common in tropical and semitropical waters. They are flat fish, with eyes on top of their body and mouths on the underside. They conceal themselves along sandy beaches to hide from prey. They use smell and electroreceptors called ampullae of Lorenzini to detect the fish, crustaceans, and mollusks that are their food source.

Stingrays have a long tail with a barbed stinger at the end. This stinger—actually a modified dermal denticle—is used for self-defense. It is about an inch long, and there are two grooves on the underside with venom glands. The stinger is covered with a thin layer of skin called the integumentary sheath, where the venom is concentrated. When the stinger breaks a human being's skin, a protein-based venom is released; sometimes the stinger breaks off and stays in the wound.

Beach lifeguards along the California coast advise swimmers to shuffle or drag their feet (do the "stingray shuffle") when they enter and exit the water, so that if they encounter a stingray, they bump it, and it swims off. If they step down on the stingray, it instinctively reacts to protect itself and may sting the swimmer.

It's also important to be aware when you're in the water. Erez Israeli, a friend of mine from Israel, decided that he wanted to start swimming in the ocean. He had swum in lakes and in the pool and traveled to Southern California to gain more experience in open water swimming. On his first ocean swim, I swam with him to see his strengths and what he needed to work on. Before we got into the water, I explained about stingrays resting and how he should slide his feet when he entered the water.

He did that, but when we were about chest-deep in the water, he was so intent on learning new information that he forgot all about the stingrays and put his feet down on the sand. Cringing, I told him that he needed to shuffle his feet to warn the stingrays that he was there, and they would swim off without bothering him. I told him about Fahmy Attallah, a long-distance swimmer, originally from Egypt, who swam off Long Beach, California, daily into his nineties. Fahmy always shuffled his feet when he entered the water. He swam breaststroke with his head above water for up to an hour a day. In all those years of swimming he had never been stung, but he didn't realize he needed to shuffle his feet when he exited the water, too.

After one morning swim, he was walking out of the water and stepped down on a stingray. When the stingray stung him, Fahmy said it was like having a hot poker stuck into his foot. His foot immediately swelled to three times its normal size, and it throbbed with pain.

A Long Beach lifeguard saw Fahmy hobbling and helped him ashore. He asked Fahmy if he was allergic to bee stings, and Fahmy told the lifeguard he wasn't. If Fahmy had shown signs of nausea, vomiting, chills, or muscle cramps, the lifeguard would have had him transported to the emergency room to be treated for an allergic reaction to the stingray venom. If Fahmy had been stung in the hand, the lifeguard would have recommended that he remove any rings or bracelets, as jewelry trapped on a swollen hand could cut off circulation.

Fahmy wasn't experiencing any signs that indicated an allergic response. The lifeguard administered first aid and had him sit down and place his foot in a bucket of water, as hot as Fahmy could tolerate. The lifeguard let the wound bleed so it would release venom from the sting and bacteria from the surrounding environment. He explained that the most intense pain came on thirty to ninety minutes after the sting, but the hot water would diminish it. (Stingray venom is composed of heat-labile proteins; hot water will alter the polypeptide protein molecule and deactivate the poison. Applying acid, such as orange juice, urine, or vinegar, does not have any effect on the sting.)

An hour later, the lifeguard applied a topical antibiotic to Fahmy's wound to reduce the chance of infection, wrapped his foot with a clean bandage, and advised him to continue soaking his foot in hot water for the next week and check the wound for signs of infection, such as redness, prolonged swelling, or pus. If this happened, he advised Fahmy to seek medical attention, as untreated infections could result in loss of limbs or death.

It took about three weeks for the swelling in Fahmy's foot to go down and the wound to heal completely. He returned to the beach and made a point of shuffling his feet when he got into the water. When he completed his workout, he swam as close to shore as he could get, splashed the water, tentatively put one foot down, and shuffled his way out of the water.

While death from stingrays is not common, Steve Irwin, an Australian television celebrity and environmentalist, was killed off the Great Barrier Reef when he swam on top of a stingray and the stingray's barb went up and into his chest and put a hole in his heart. An important reminder: When you're in the open water, keep in mind that you're swimming with wild animals. It is best to keep a safe distance.

WATER ENTRY

Nick Bolin, in addition to being a lifeguard, is a surfer, triathlete, and open water swimmer. He is in tune with the ocean. He offered the following observations and insights: "The ocean is dynamic, fluid, and always changing. In a matter of hours, water conditions can go from what appears to be very calm and gentle to turbulent seas. Ocean conditions are affected by a variety of different things, such as water temperature, tides, surf, bottom contour, sandbars, wind, and currents, just to name a few. It is always a good idea to check with your local lifeguard agency before entering the water."

Lifeguards are trained to spot rip currents and trouble-some areas and can point swimmers in the direction where it is safest to swim. It is always recommended to swim at a beach that is guarded. Talk with the lifeguards and let them know your swim plan and how long you plan to be out. Be open to the lifeguard's suggestions; some areas may be closed to swimming, while others have limits on how far a swimmer can venture out. These limits are placed for safety reasons. Variables such as vessel traffic and other water sports may be harmful to a swimmer.

For the beginning open water swimmer: Start on a beach with very little or no surf. You can gradually work your way into surf conditions, but remember that even open water with little or no tide is a lot different from swimming in a pool. It is always advised to swim with a buddy or a group. If you are new to open water swimming, go with someone experienced who can help you get com-fortable in the new environment.

Nick Bolin offered the following recommendations for entering the water:

~ Enter slowly, and never dive headfirst.
~ If you need to get under a wave, always keep your hands out in front of you.
~ Wait for a lull in the surf to enter the water. (A lull is the calm between wave sets.)
~ Swim through the surf impact zone quickly to get to the "outside," where waves are not breaking.

It never occurred to me why it was so crucial to enter and exit the water this way until years later, when I heard about a new junior guard who forgot to extend his arms over his head while bodysurfing to shore. A wave slammed him into the beach, and he lost all use of his arms and legs.

The United States Lifesaving Association recommends the following steps to avoid spinal injury:

~ Swim near a lifeguard.

~ Check with lifeguards about current conditions before swimming.

~ Stop, watch, and walk into the water.

~ Don't dive headfirst into any unknown water.

~ Don't dive toward the bottom into oncoming waves.

~ Don't stand with your back to the waves.

~ Don't jump or dive from a cliff, pier, jetty, or bridge.

~ Avoid bodysurfing, body boarding, or surfing straight "over the falls." Ride the shoulder.

~ In a "wipeout," land as flat as possible with your hands out in front of you.

~ While bodysurfing, keep an arm out in front of you to protect your head and neck.

~ When in doubt, *don't dive*—play it safe!

BODYSURFING

Bodysurfing and bobbing in waves are what first attracted me into the cold Atlantic waters. Dave, my brother, and I bodysurfed along the New England coast into narrow sandy beaches framed by enormous rocks and rugged peninsulas where waves broke like thunder and water sprayed sky-high. We loved the feeling of the white water breaking around our legs, the sudden lift and bounce of the water, the awesome power and beauty of the funneling waves, and the deep chill of the dark blue ocean.

As children, Dave and my two sisters, Laura and Ruth, and I bodysurfed in small one- and two-foot waves. As teenagers, we spent our free time bodysurfing in the Pacific Ocean along Long Beach, Seal Beach, and Huntington Beach.

We asked surfers for tips, like how we could extend our fun by extending our rides. We asked them what to do when we were held down by big wave sets. They told us to relax and hang out underwater until the large set passed. We asked them what to do when we got spun around under the water and couldn't tell which direction was up. They told us to follow our bubbles back to the surface.

For those who are starting out with open water swimming, it is important to get good instruction on-site from local lifeguards, surfers, and experienced open water swimmers. They study the waves and know when it is safe to go and when it is not. They also will tell you where you don't want to be in the surf zone.

Bodysurfing is like starts and turns in pool swimming. The speed at which you enter and exit the water can determine whether you win a race or get safely off- or onshore.

Thinking about the SEALs and their ability to handle all kinds of water conditions, I asked L. Tadeus if the trainees have any special training for going through the surf. He explained what the SEALs do:

~ Many of the SEAL trainees have a surfing background. They go through the surf with a buddy, and they have instructors who are lifeguards, watching them get through the surf zone.

~ When going through the surf zone, ideally, a swimmer should swim beneath the wave about two to three feet and keep breaststroking forward to get himself past the plunging wave faster. The surfing term for this is "duck diving." The reason we teach this is because water is fairly incompressible, and most of the turbulence from the wave action—regardless of wave size—is limited to the first couple of feet below the plunging wave. You still feel a surge of water, but not the washing machine effect.

~ If a swimmer is caught by a wave, certainly, curling up and protecting the head is warranted—in fact, recommended, especially in the case of coral reefs under really heavy surf.

~ The trick is to protect your head and core from major impact damage and, in the case of a diver, from the equipment being worn.

WAVES

Waves are part of what makes open water swimming very different from pool swimming. They make open water swimming more fun and more challenging than swimming in a predictable swimming pool. Waves also make the swimmer stronger and more aware of and connected to the environment.

According to the NOAA National Weather Service, waves are created by three components: wind strength, as the wind must be moving faster than the wave crests for energy to be transferred; wind duration, since a strong wind that does not blow for a long period will not generate large waves; and wind fetch, the uninterrupted distance over which the wind blows without significant change in direction. An interesting aside: The Pacific Ocean has the largest uninterrupted water surface, so waves in the Pacific can grow larger than in any of the other oceans in the world.

After the wind has blown for a period of time, the waves grow higher from the trough (the bottom of the wave) to the crest (the top of the wave), and both the wavelength and wave period (the time interval between the arrival of consecutive crests at a stationary point) become longer. As the wind continues blowing or strengthening in force, the water first forms whitecaps, and then the waves break. This is known as a fully developed sea.

The waves in a fully developed sea move faster than the storm that creates them, lengthening and reducing in height in the process. These are called swell waves. Swells organize into groups that are smooth and regular in appearance. They are able to travel thousands of miles unchanged in height and wave period.

The longer the wave, the faster it travels. As waves leave storm areas, they tend to sort themselves out with the long ones ahead of the short ones, and the energy is simultaneously spread out over an increasingly larger area. As the waves close in on the coast, they begin to feel the bottom, and their direction of travel might change due to the contour of the land. Eventually, the waves run ashore, increasing in height up to one and a half times their height in deep water, finally breaking up as surf.

Getting in and out of the impact zone is one of the most important considerations when open water swimming.

SURF

Sean Collins, formerly the president, chief surf forecaster, and founder of Surfline, a worldwide source for wave forecasting, spent most of his life surfing the world's big waves and sailing across the great oceans. Through these experiences, he thoroughly studied weather systems, their movements, and when and where the storm systems would generate winds and surf.

Over the past twenty-five years, Sean honed his research and observation skills and developed a sophisticated proprietary system of wave forecasting, much of which is currently used in LOLA, Surfline's global swell model.

These wave forecasts are available at Surfline.com. Surfline has provided weather and forecasting services to every lifeguard agency in California, the Coast Guard, U.S. Navy SEALs, the National Weather Service, numerous television and movie production companies, multiple domestic and international governmental agencies, and nearly every surf company in the world.

Sean was a pioneer in surf monitoring and developed the first live "surfcam" in 1996, the precedent for the famous camera network available on Surfline.com today. In July 2008, Sean was inducted into the Surfers' Hall of

Fame, with his footprints and handprints immortalized in stone on the corner of Pacific Coast Highway and Main Street in Huntington Beach.

Sean was the source of big wave forecasts for the big wave riders, including Mike Parsons, Brad Gerlach, Shane Dorian, Laird Hamilton, Greg and Rusty Long, Jamie Sterling, and many more. Sean surfed and explored waves by land, air, and sea for over forty years. He passed his knowledge on to his son, and they spent their time together surfing in the secret surf spot south of the border. In the spirit of sharing his knowledge with others, Sean provided the following guidelines for swimmers who are planning to swim in the ocean:

~ Before swimmers go to the beach, they should check the surf report and see if there is surf. You can check with Surfline.com and the National Weather Service.
~ Talk with the lifeguards about the surf before you get in the water.
~ Watch the water for fifteen minutes before you enter. Look out at the waves. Look in front of the wave break close to shore. Look right at the wave break, and look outside the waves; the current is different in every one of these areas, and the current is different every day.

Sean cautioned, "One of the most dangerous areas in the ocean is the surf zone. It's where you have multiple forces meeting. You have surf compressing against shallow water and sand, and you have currents near shore, and they are stronger in the surf zone. Everything in the surf zone is being compressed against the hard surface of the sand. You will also have the surf beat, where the water is being trapped on the beach. This water has to escape and flow out, and this creates another current."

Sean was describing a rip current, which can carry a swimmer far offshore. How to get out of one will be discussed shortly, but Sean recommends first knowing how to identify a rip current in order to avoid it:

~ Watch how the water is moving and how it is traveling from one area to another.
~ Watch the water fifty feet from shore and find pieces of kelp, foam, things that float in, and see how they move or don't move.
~ Look farther out and see how these telltales are moving.
~ Walk the beach before you swim and watch the water and how it moves.

Rip currents can also be used as an advantage. SEALs note where the rips are occurring and use them to assist through the surf zone. They also use rips to take boats through the "boat zone." They have found that many people who drown in the ocean do so because they find themselves being pushed out to sea, then swim against this current until they tire out completely and succumb. The remedy to this situation is to swim perpendicularly until you are out of the rip.

Sean added, "The ocean is magical. Everything is constantly changing. The secret is to see what the ocean is trying to communicate to you, and you recognize it, and you adjust to the ocean's mood. It is important to understand what is happening in the ocean before you get in the water. You can't count on someone saving you; you need to anticipate what the changing conditions will be. Think about how things are going to change during your swim, before you even start, so you will be able to react to the water."

ROLE OF THE TIDES

Sean Collins explained the way the tides affect the surf and the route of your swims: "Tides are connected to the moon and sun. Tidal currents are strongest near an inlet or bay. It's important to understand when it is high tide and when the highest high or the lowest low will occur. This happens in the middle of the tide, not at the end of a tide. If the water movement is very strong, it will push you way off course or out of the bay. You need to know what the water is doing before you get in."

Sean advised using certain signs and telltales as references:

~ If you are trying to figure out what the wind will be doing, look at the freighters offshore. They are always pointed into the wind.
~ The wind usually starts offshore from a higher altitude. Look at the treetops and flagpoles, and you will be able to forecast which direction the wind will blow across the water. Think of air as you would water. A high-pressure area will flow to a low-pressure area to equalize itself, just like water moves to equalize itself.

Sean has observed nature and studied charts to create forecasts; he has also used his hearing. He said, "I figured out that where there is a high-pressure area moving in, the sounds you hear around you make a small echo. You hear that echo and know that a high-pressure system is on land. The winds die, and the waves get really good. The high-pressure systems press down on the land and cause the sound waves to change."

SWELL PREDICTION

From Sean's kitchen window, we watched the surf breaking along the shores of Seal Beach. For four or five different swells, Sean observed the angle they hit the beach, the size of the waves, and the time between the waves. In this way, Sean could tell where the waves originated. He tracked the origin of storms and their movements around the world. Based on the speed of the storm's movement and the energy the wind put into the water in the form of waves, Sean could tell from the angles at which the waves hit the beach, and by the time between the waves, where each wave came from. Each wave had its own unique fingerprint, Sean said. He saw two waves hit the beach and said they came from a storm off Fiji, and then he saw one coming from a storm off Hawaii.

Sean gave the following directions for entering the surf zone:

~ Watch the waves break.
~ Surf comes in sets, and there are calm periods in between, known as lulls.
~ Time your entry or exit during the lull period.
~ Big lulls occur between big sets of waves.
~ Understand ocean-floor contours. Waves break because they are moving over shallow water. Waves rise up, become unstable, and break.

L. Tadeus noted another surfer rule of thumb: Waves break twice as high as the water is deep. The wave may break, then fade briefly, then break again as it moves over the contours of the ocean floor. Understanding underwater hydrography is exceedingly important to any competent waterman.

To understand the way the water is moving, Sean suggested that you:

~ Watch some waves break. It is usually better to swim through deep water than shallow water, but watch beforehand to make sure there isn't a lot of current in the deep-water areas.
~ Talk to fishermen about the currents. Fish like currents. Where there is current, the fish start to feed. Fish have a great sense of smell. They start smelling other fish when

there is current. The current takes the scent and moves it around. Fishermen are tuned into tides and currents.
~ Talk to the pros who are on the water every day.
~ Figure out the current and watch the surf line, the winds, and the waves.
~ Don't let something happen and then have to figure out what to do. Be aware before you swim.

MOVING THROUGH THE SURF

Nick Bolin offered additional advice for getting through the surf zone.

~ Look ahead to see the approaching waves/set.
~ If a wave breaks right in front of you or a wall of white-wash is coming at you, take a deep breath and swim toward the bottom. This allows the swimmer to get underneath the breaking wave.
~ Once the wave passes, return to the surface. Look ahead to see if other waves are approaching.
~ Try to make your way through the surf zone quickly. Once you're on the outside area of the breaking waves, it is generally much calmer.

OVER OUR HEADS: DISTRESS SIGNALS

The ocean changes rapidly. Even though we try to get the best information before we swim, and make the best judgments, sometimes we need some help. There is nothing wrong with asking for help. It is far better to be embarrassed and avoid getting hurt.

There are certain distress signals to let lifeguards know that you are in trouble or in need of assistance.

~ Call out for help.
~ Wave your arms to gather attention.
~ Relax; try not to panic.
~ Don't fight the current.

RIPTIDES

Before you swim, check with the NOAA/National Weather Service for surf zone forecasts. They will contain information about potential riptides in the area where you'll be swimming. NOAA has a listing of rip currents called "Rip Current Outlooks," listing the risk from low to high:

~ Low risk of rip currents: Wind and/or wave conditions are not strong enough to create rip currents.
~ Moderate risk of rip currents: Wind and/or wave conditions support stronger or more frequent rip currents. Only experienced surf swimmers should enter the water.
~ High risk of rip currents: Wind and/or wave conditions support dangerous rip currents. Rip currents are life threatening to anyone entering the surf. Rip currents may be moderate or high risks, especially in the areas around jetties and piers.
~ When you arrive at the beach, speak with on-duty lifeguards about rip currents and all other water conditions expected for the day.

NOAA also advises:

~ Know the meaning of and obey warnings represented by colored beach flags.
~ Take your cell phone to the beach. In case of an emergency, if the lifeguard is not present, call 911.

Different beaches may use different colors, but here is a commonly used series:

~ Double red: beach is closed to the public.
~ Single red: high hazard; for example, strong surf or currents.
~ Yellow: medium hazard.
~ Green: calm conditions, although caution is still necessary.
~ Purple (flown with either red or yellow): dangerous marine life but not sharks.

Ways to Identify a Riptide

You can often spot the areas where there are riptides. They typically happen when a lot of surf piles up on the beach and the water needs to flow back into the ocean. You will see areas of discolored sandy water that are roughly ten to fifty feet wide and flowing out into the ocean. They look like small streams of murky water.

~ Before you get into the water, ask the lifeguard about the conditions.
~ Never swim alone.
~ Never swim at night. Rip currents can be more dangerous at night simply because you cannot see them.
~ Stay at least a hundred feet away from piers and jetties. Permanent rip currents often exist alongside these structures.

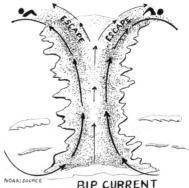

NOAA: SOURCE

RIP CURRENT

~ Use polarized sunglasses. They will help you to spot signatures of rip currents by cutting down glare and sunlight reflected off the ocean's surface.

~ Avoid the "it won't/didn't happen to me" syndrome. Obey all instructions/orders from lifeguards and posted signs.

Caught in a Rip

~ Remain calm. You will not be pulled under the surface of the water.

~ Swim parallel to the shore only to escape the current. As soon as you are out of the current, only then swim toward the beach. Do not swim directly against the current. It will be too strong for you.

~ Another option is to float. Eventually, you will reach the end of the current. Then either:

~ Swim parallel to the shore to get out of the path of the rip current and, once you do so, only then swim toward the beach; or:

~ Draw attention to yourself by waving your arms and yelling for help (which you can do because you are not swimming alone ... right?).

WATER EXIT

After you've completed a workout, if you've worked hard, you're tired, but you need to concentrate and be aware of what the surf is doing so you know how get in to shore.

Nick Bolin offered the following advice regarding exiting the water:

~ As you swim toward the shore, check behind you to see if there are waves. Try to determine the depth of the water if possible, as that can be indicative of when the waves will start breaking. Swim a couple of strokes on your back, or stop and look back to see if there are approaching waves.

~ It is possible to catch a wave and ride it in to the shore. Although bodysurfing may look easy, it is actually more difficult than it looks. You must be swimming at a good rate of speed to catch a wave just as it is breaking and have a chance of riding it in. Most important, if you are attempting to catch a wave, make sure your hands are out in front of you at all times. A shallow spot or sand-bar may present itself at any moment. By keeping your hands out in front, you are protecting your head and neck from slamming into the ocean bottom.

~ Sometimes conditions are rough and not conducive to wave riding. As when you enter the water, you may have to take a deep breath, swim toward the bottom, and let the wave pass over the top of you. By not swimming deep enough or coming up too early, swimmers jeopar-dize themselves and get caught in the wave. The wave will pick you up, sometimes referred to as going over the falls or getting caught in the washing machine cycle.

If you go over the falls, L. Tadeus said, "I recommend curling into a ball, because: 1. If you are near coral reefs, extending extremities can get wedged between coral heads though your body is still moving (ouch); 2. Balling up pro-tects the head and core as you tumble across the bottom; 3. You get out of the washing machine faster because you expose less 'sail' area to the water action. The safest way to go through the surf is duck diving—doing a shallow dive under the wave."

Most important, keep an eye out to sea as you near the shore. Start with small surf and work into larger surf as your comfort and swim level allow. If you are unsure about going out, then don't. Surf varies from beach to beach. Although one beach may be experiencing a large swell, a lot of times you can drive just a few miles and find another area with smaller surf.

For more information about safe swimming in the ocean, water conditions, and up-to-date news, check out the American Lifeguard Association or the United States Lifesaving Association. The United States Lifeguard Association has a training manual that they use to instruct beach lifeguards. The manual is full of helpful health and safety information. See Sources for each organization's website address; page 300.

Chapter 7

Effects of Heat and Cold

For over thirty years, I've been involved in research on cold acclimatization and hypothermia. Researchers, physicians, and physiologists at the University of California, Santa Barbara, in the Institute of Environmental Stress, began studying my ability to acclimate to cold during my freshman year of college. Their objectives were to discover how people acclimate to the cold, to find better ways to recover from cold exposure, and to increase survival time in cold environments. They had done a number of heat studies on world-class marathon runners, including Jackie Hansen, a world record holder. The scientists said that most people would not volunteer to be in cold studies.

They knew that I had trained with Don Gambril, who had coached the U.S. Olympic team, and that I had swum across the English and Catalina Channels and had broken the men's and women's world records, and they thought I had somehow acclimated to the cold. They also knew that I was training to become the first person to swim across the Strait of Magellan.

The team of researchers believed that what they discovered from studying me could help people survive in the cold. They wanted to develop better methods for rewarming people, and to know how the human body acclimated to the cold. They also said that their studies would contribute to basic medical research. They thought that, through their studies, physicians might find better ways to cool people for heart surgery, as well as ways to use the cold to reduce inflammation from head and spinal injury. In return, they would teach me advanced physiology that might help me with my open water swimming goals.

The team of researchers—led by Dr. Steven Horvath, Dr. Barbara Drinkwater, Dr. William McCafferty, and graduate student Annie Loucks—and a group of physicians and graduate students began conducting a series of studies on me in cold rooms at the institute, in a cold tank of water, and before and after my cold-water training swims off the shores of Goleta, California. What they observed surprised them.

COLD ACCLIMATIZATION

When most people swim in cold water, they pump the warm blood from their core to their extremities. The blood in the extremities is not as insulated as it is in the core, and it absorbs cold from the surrounding water. When the blood from the extremities circulates back to the core, body temperature drops. The researchers found that I responded differently to the cold. I was able to keep the blood in the core of my body instead of pumping it out to my extremities. They saw that I had a well-distributed layer of body fat that helped to insulate my body and keep my core warm; plus, I was in great shape and able to swim for miles at 70 to 80 percent of my maximum physical ability because I had worked with some of the top coaches in the world, including my older brother, Dave. During the intense physical workouts, my body created more heat than it lost.

This cold research gained the attention of Dr. William R. Keatinge, the world's expert on hypothermia. He was visiting the research team at UCSB when they introduced him to me. He began doing a series of blood flow and infrared studies on me at the University of London.

The researchers at UCSB and University of London discovered that my body had acclimated to the cold. They had me swim tethered in a 42-degree F (5.5-degree C) tank of cold water and monitored me. After a four-hour swim in 50-degree F (10-degree C) water, my core temperature increased to 102.2 degrees F (39 degrees C). The researchers were astonished. We repeated the test four times to confirm the findings.

The scientists were extremely excited. This acclimatization process was something that had been observed by the great Norwegian polar explorers Fridtjof Nansen, the first European to cross the frigid Greenland ice cap; and Roald Amundsen, the first man to reach the brutally cold South Pole. They understood it over a hundred years ago. In order to cross the Greenland ice cap or reach the South Pole, they needed to train and sleep in cold environments to acclimate. Their conditioning made all the difference.

On his crossing of the Greenland ice cap, Nansen experienced 70 degrees below F (56.6 degrees below C). The air inside his reindeer tent was so cold that it fogged with his breath, and the condensation of his breath turned to ice on his beard. Amundsen emulated Nansen: He skied during the long cold Norwegian winters and slept with his bedroom window open at times when temperatures plummeted to 40 degrees below F (40 degrees below C). They endured temperatures that most humans have never experienced.

Acclimating to the cold water has taken me many years of intense training and increased exposure to the cold, as well as a gradual drop in cold-water temperatures. My coldest swim to date was in May 2007, off the shores of Disko Bay, Greenland, where the water temperature ranged from 26.6 to 28.8 degrees F (3 degrees below to 1.8 degrees C) and I swam a quarter of a mile in five minutes and ten seconds.

Brownie Schoene, a Wilderness Medicine physician, pulmonary specialist, researcher, and friend helped me prepare for swims that had never been done before. He told me how differently unacclimated people respond to cold water. During a trip to Antarctica, Brownie was the ship's physician. He recounted a story about three men in a Zodiac who fell overboard in 32- to 33-degree F (0 to 1 degree C) water. Brownie said one man stayed by the Zodiac boat. The second man swam halfway back to the ship, about one hundred yards, before he was picked up by a support boat. The third man swam about two hundred yards to the ship.

The ship's medics cared for the victims and, in their evaluations, measured the temperatures of the individuals and discovered that the man with the highest core temperature was the one who had stayed beside the Zodiac, curled up in a ball; the man who was halfway back to the ship had a lower core temperature; and the man who swam all the way back to the ship had the lowest core temperature. None of them had trained in water, and none had acclimated to the cold. As a result, their body temperatures dropped rapidly in the cold water, but the one who had exposed less of his body's surface area to the cold water underwent the least loss of body heat. In other words, the potent convective force of the flow of very cold water, which wicks away heat, had the greatest effect on those who tried to swim. Brownie said that this event provided cogent lessons in both optimizing survival as well as thermal physiology. These results are consistent with those who swam farther having more blood flow to the arms and legs, more heat loss, and thus, greater decrease in core temperature. It also underscored the need for swimmers to acclimate to cold water.

My process for acclimating to the cold began at age fourteen, when a group of teenagers invited me to swim across the Catalina Channel. My father, a physician, knew about cold acclimatization and advised us to train in cool waters, to wear light clothing and sandals, and to sleep with our bedroom windows open. This would condition our bodies to cooler environments. The water temperature was in the high sixties when we swam across the Catalina Channel, and I learned that if you are not swimming at your normal speed and creating heat, you will gradually lose heat and be cold throughout the swim.

After the Catalina Channel, my goal became the English Channel. At first I trained in the Pacific, in water temperatures ranging from 50 to 70 degrees F (10 to 20 degrees C), and in swimming pools that were between 76 to 78 degrees F (24.4 to 25.5 degrees C).

Quickly, it became evident that training in a swimming pool did not help me acclimate to the cold water. During my training swims in the pool, my face turned bright red, and sweat streamed down my face; my body was overheating. I decided to train only in the ocean. At ages fifteen and sixteen, I swam across the English Channel and broke the men's and women's world records twice. Many people who attempt the English Channel have problems staying warm. Some have gone into hypothermia—a body temperature below 95 degrees F (35 degrees C)—and a handful of swimmers have died from hypothermia when their core temperature dropped too far. The way I had acclimated enabled me to swim in the cool waters of the English Channel. Not everyone can acclimate to the cold. Some do it better than others, and some can acclimate to heat, while others can't. I am not good at swimming in warm or hot waters; I overheat.

Heat is an equally important consideration in open water swimming. Just as hypothermia (a lowered core body temperature) is dangerous for swimmers, so, too, is hyperthermia (a high core temperature).

HYPERTHERMIA AND HYPOTHERMIA

Hyperthermia and hypothermia are two potentially life-threatening conditions that swimmers can experience if they have not acclimated. Hyperthermia is defined as a dangerously high core temperature, and hypothermia is a dangerously low core temperature.

Because hyperthermia and hypothermia may affect swimmers' judgment during their swims, they may not realize that they are in danger. It is very important to have a safety person on the support boat who can recognize the symptoms of hypothermia or hyperthermia—which include shivering, purple lips, splayed fingers, purple shoulders, disorientation, and confusion—and tell the swimmer that he or she must stop. Swimmers experiencing hyperthermia or hypothermia cannot be relied upon to be their own voice of reason.

Hyperthermia is a body temperature greater than 101.3 degrees F (38.5 degrees C). It occurs when the person's body produces or absorbs more heat than it can give off, whereupon the heat-regulating mechanisms of the body become overwhelmed and are not able to expel excess heat. This may cause body temperature to climb uncontrollably. It is a medical emergency, and the individual should get immediate medical treatment to prevent injury or death.

In severe cases, the person's temperature can exceed 104 degrees F (40 degrees C). Significant physical exertion on a very hot day or swimming in hot tropical waters can generate heat beyond a healthy person's ability to cool himself or herself, since heat and humidity reduce the efficiency of the body's normal cooling mechanisms (such as vasodilation and sweating). During strenuous exercise, heat production in the body is increased ten to twenty times.

This is something to be aware of when swimming in warm water. Fran Crippen, an Olympic silver medalist and one of the world's top open water swimmers, died of hyperthermia during an international competition off the shores of Dubai. He overheated during the race, but no one noticed that he was in trouble. Fran recognized the critical importance of having an adequate number of support boats, kayakers, and safety crew to watch over the swimmers during the race, but sadly, his suggestions were not followed. His death made officials examine the cause of his death and ways to implement more safety measures to make people aware of the possibility of hyperthermia during open water swimming and how to prevent it.

Sweating and vasodilatation are the major mechanisms of heat loss to maintain your body core temperature. Dr. Gordon Giesbrecht, an expert in environmental stress at the University of Manitoba, explained,

Hyperthermia is caused by increased heat production through exercise in a warm/hot, often humid environment. As ambient temperature increases, the temperature gradient for heat to be lost from the body decreases, and body heat builds up. The purpose of sweating is to provide a fluid that can evaporate from the body surface or within the contacting layers of clothes. The process of evaporation (changing the state of liquid from liquid to gas) requires energy; therefore, evaporation from the skin or clothing takes heat away from the body. As humidity rises, the water content rises, and the ability of sweat to evaporate diminishes. At later stages of heat illness, victims also lose the ability to sweat because of severe dehydration, and of course heat continues to build up and core temperature rises.

L. Tadeus said,

We cool trainees if they get above 102 degrees F (38.8 degrees C). Anything above 105 degrees F (40.5 degrees C) is our threshold for a medical emergency. Core temperatures of 107 degrees F (41.6 degrees C) can result in death. I'm talking about *ice bath*—not sitting in an air-conditioned room. Our trainees do not reenter the training pipeline after a heat/cold injury without successfully completing a heat stress test and being cleared by our medical staff.

Gordon Giesbrecht added, "There is evidence that you might have an increased risk of heat illness once you have overheated. There is also evidence that you might have an increased risk of local cold injury (i.e., frostbite or non-freezing cold injury [NFCI] after a cold injury). There is less evidence that you have increased risk of hypothermia, certainly not at the mild to moderate level."

HEAT ACCLIMATIZATION

One of the ways to prevent hyperthermia is to acclimate to the heat. According to the Navy Environmental Health Center Bureau of Medicine Health Center:

Acclimatization is a process of physiologic adaptation to heat stress conditions. After acclimatization, a person's tolerance of and performance in heat stress conditions are improved.

Acclimatization is accomplished by exposure to heat stress over a period of days or weeks. Exposure to heat for one hour or less, even with exercise, will not accomplish the acclimatization. It is possible only with longer daily exposures.

Heat acclimatization occurs more rapidly in persons with greater cardiopulmonary fitness. Active women may acclimatize to heat at a faster rate or to a greater extent than active men. Physical conditioning is also advantageous in the body's response to dehydration, a heat stress—related condition. In one study, physical conditioning was associated with enhanced work performance during dehydration.

Inactivity results in decreased acclimatization after only a few days or weeks. Exposing heat-acclimatized individuals regularly to cold temperatures can cause a significant loss in heat acclimatization. A single exercise and/or heat exposure per week was no different from complete cessation of endurance exercise in the heat with regard to loss of acclimatization-related changes in plasma volume. Acclimatization-related changes in sweat gland function may be attenuated by increases in central dopaminergic activity.

I learned from Dr. Keatinge that if you're acclimated to the cold, you won't acclimate well to the heat. Your body can't do both at the same time.

Gordon Giesbrecht suggested starting early, "well before you plan to swim in warm or hot water; gradually building up to the work and thermal stress; and getting to know your body." He said, "Don't just go out and do it and try to power through it. You'll lose. You need to take a lot of time, and you need to monitor your responses. Make adjustments according to how you're feeling, and swim with a buddy who knows you and knows when you are doing well and when you aren't. The more you understand this process, the more you'll be able to figure out what works for you and what doesn't."

SEAL Hyperthermia Experiences

Because the SEALs work in environments of extreme hot and cold, I asked L. Tadeus if he'd ever experienced hyperthermia or hypothermia. He recounted his experience with hyperthermia:

My platoon was training in the desert more than a decade ago, and even at night the temperature was over 95 degrees F (35 degrees C). Our objective was to practice patrolling to a location, then construct a "spider hole," and finally lay up in this location to observe a logistical line of communication and report what we saw via satellite to a rear echelon tactical operation center (TOC).

We had to dig into the sand and backfill the hole with sandbags to stabilize the walls. We would then cover the hole with tarp and sand so that it appeared nothing had changed. Three of us manned the position as the sun came up, and the rest of the platoon patrolled back to base. We were already beat, dehydrated, and pretty much angry at the universe when the sun came up.

After we'd spent all day in the hole, the inside started to swelter, and I and another member of the three-man element became increasingly dehydrated. We were drinking as much as we could but were already behind the power curve.

The senior man in the hole made the decision to call for a MEDEVAC, and the training cadre came to our location with a van to pick us up. We were ordered to break down our position, fill in the hole we'd dug, and prepare to return.

My fellow victim and I had all the classic symptoms: We had both stopped sweating. Even when we were standing in midday sun in 120 degrees F (48.8 degrees C) heat, the slightest breeze felt really cool. As we broke down our position, we were emptying sandbags. Every time I bent down to empty a sandbag, I would get very dizzy—it felt like when you squat down for a while, then stand back up and get a little light-headed, only times ten. I would need to sit down and rest for a minute or so after each sandbag. This was, of course, due to severely low blood pressure brought on by dehydration. We were both extremely lethargic. It felt like time was slowing down a bit. My ears were ringing, I was getting a little bit of tunnel vision, and I felt dissociated from events happening around me. I can only describe the feeling as surreal—it was like everyone's voice around me was echoing inside my head.

When we returned to the training compound, we were both given a once-over by the docs. I still can't figure out why nobody ever got our rectal temperatures. My partner was so dehydrated that his veins had collapsed and intravenous fluids were not an option. It took the docs about ten minutes to find a workable vein in my arm. After about ten sticks, they finally got a good vein. I took about five bags of fluid over the next few hours, and my partner drank water until he could urinate, which took a few hours. We both had a huge hangover the next morning and flulike soreness over our entire bodies for the whole day.

I can only assume our core temps were somewhere in the 105-degree F (41.8 degrees C) range, based on my experience with hyperthermia as a trainer.

We recently had a trainee go down with hyperthermia. He was participating in a four-mile timed run. As always, there is not only pressure to pass but also to exceed their previous score. The trainee had just returned from a two-week holiday stand-down, and this was his first run since returning. The time standard is 4 miles (6.4 kilometers) in 31 minutes, a little less than an 8-minute mile and definitely not a world-record pace.

This trainee was set to meet the standard but was near the back of the pack. However, about two hundred meters from the finish line, he collapsed. He was assessed within fifteen seconds or so by the on-scene medical staff, then placed in the emergency vehicle and transported to a medical facility that was nearby.

His core temperature was taken with a rectal probe and discovered to be at 107.5 degrees F (41.9 degrees C), which is about as close to death by overheating as you can get. He was immediately bathed in ice, given intravenous fluids, and assessed until his core temperature dropped below 102 degrees F (38.8 degrees C).

He exhibited many of the same symptoms. He was able to power through the lethargy by sheer force of will and by adjusting his run technique—he was throwing his whole body into it. He had stopped sweating a little over halfway through the run. He remembered nothing about the run after the two-mile turnaround point. He was very lethargic and incoherent between the time of his collapse and his arrival at a treatment facility.

His core temp was so high that he probably cooked a few brain cells. It was also so high that he had to be assessed forty-five days after the incident, using heat-stress tests to ensure that his susceptibility to further heat injuries did not physically disqualify him from the program.

~ Water heats the body twenty-five times faster than air at the same temperature.
~ Make sure to drink enough water while exercising in warm to hot water. Hot air can make hyperthermia worse.

Symptoms of Heat Exhaustion

Normal to slightly elevated core temperature.

Fatigue or malaise.

Orthostatic hypotension (dizzy when standing up), tachycardia (rapid heart rate, over 100 beats per minute).

Clinical signs of dehydration.

Nausea, vomiting, diarrhea.

Mental confusion.

Treatment for Heat Exhaustion

Place in a tub of cool water.

Give fluid and electrolyte replacement.

Symptoms of Heatstroke

Elevated core temperature, usually greater than 104.9 degrees F (40.5 degrees C).

Weakness, nausea, vomiting, headache.

Central nervous system symptoms, including confusion, not able to be stable on feet, coma, seizures, delirium.

Loss of ability to sweat, resulting in hot, dry skin.

Fever.

Shivering.

Treatment for Heatstroke

Call 911.

Pour as much water as possible on the victim's head and fan air over the victim as much as possible (either with an electric fan or manually). Clothing will trap the water against the skin until it evaporates and takes heat from the body. If the victim's clothes are removed, much of the water poured on the victim will merely roll off onto the ground and not participate in heat loss.

If the victim is not wearing much clothing, apply the water more to the shorts and shirt than bare areas.

Wet washcloths with cool water and place on the victim's forehead and body.

Immerse victim in cold or ice water.

HYPOTHERMIA

Gordon Giesbrecht said that hypothermia is clinically defined when core temperature decreases from normal to below 95 degrees F (35 degrees C). Mild hypothermia is from 95 to 90 degrees F (35 to 32 degrees C); moderate hypothermia is from 90 to 82 degrees F (32 to 28 degrees C); and severe hypothermia is below 82 degrees F (below 38 degrees C). This physical condition needs treatment when body temperature falls below 95 degrees F (35 degrees C). Hypothermia becomes life threatening when body temperature drops below 90 degrees F (32.2 degrees C).

Any decrease in core temperature (for example, above 95 degrees F—35 degrees C—and thus not clinically hypothermic) indicates that there is some uncompensated heat loss and that core temperature will likely continue to drop unless something changes (such as increasing heat production/delivery and/or decreased heat loss). The initial signs of cold stress are feeling cold and shivering, a heat production mechanism that normally occurs to prevent hypothermia in the first place. The "umbles" is a simple pneumonic that can be used to remember the early stages of hypothermia (from *Hypothermia, Frostbite and other Cold Injuries* by Gordon Giesbrecht and David Wilkerson, Mountain Books, Seattle, 2006):

Fumbles: Small muscle groups get cold and fine motor control is lost.

Stumbles: Large muscle groups get cold and gross motor control is affected.

Tumbles: The victim is unable to walk or stand.

Grumbles: Early on, the victim is irritable.

Mumbles: Further cooling affects brain function and talking is difficult.

A decrease in mental function leads to impaired ability to make decisions. A swimmer may appear tired, lethargic, disoriented, and slur words or have other changes in speech. The person may appear drunk.

As people get older, their shivering reflex diminishes (in the moderate to severe range), and the defense heat production mechanism is less effective. People experiencing hypothermia may become unable to walk or stand and eventually lose consciousness (this occurs somewhere between 90 to 86 degrees F, or 32 to 30 degrees C).

Although there used to be a belief that warming a cold victim pre-hospital was dangerous, there is now general agreement that moderate warming of a patient in the field or during pre-hospital transport (anything short of putting the patient in a warm bath or shower) is beneficial and safe. The main priorities of treatment are to remove the victim from the cold stress; halt the decrease in core temperature; maintain cardiovascular stability; and support steady, safe core rewarming, as indicated by the Alaska State Guidelines for Treatment of Hypothermia, Frostbite, and other Cold Injury. The concern was that pre-hospital warming would cause massive vasodilation, cardiovascular collapse, and death. However, the only way that can happen is if a victim is placed in a tub of warm/hot water or in a warm/ hot shower. Thus, a victim should *never be placed* in a tub of warm or hot water. Any other type of warming available to pre-hospital personnel is safe. These treatments include: chemical, electric, or charcoal heat packs; warm water bottles (rigid or flexible); skin-to-skin body-to-body contact; warm water–perfused or electric blankets.

A victim should be gently removed from danger and then moved to a sheltered area, keeping the victim as horizontal as possible. Rough handling can induce ventricular fibrillation, and vertical position can cause decreased blood pressure (due to blood pooling in the legs) and increased after-drop in core temperature (as blood flows to the cold limbs and returns to the heart). Any wet clothing should be removed (by cutting it off) and the victim dried by blotting, not rubbing, and then placed in as much insulation as possible.

A mildly hypothermic patient will be conscious and shivering vigorously. This shivering will eventually warm the core, so external heat is not necessary. However, external heat does attenuate shivering, and thus the work of the heart, providing more comfort. A moderately to severely hypothermic patient—who will have weak or no shivering and diminished or no consciousness—should be actively warmed by whatever means is available (except any form of water bath or shower). Once the patient is in a stable enclosure, transfer to hospital should ensue immediately.

SEAL Hypothermia Experiences

L. Tadcus recounted his experience of hypothermia and the experiences of some SEAL trainees:

My platoon was conducting cold-water dive training in the Pacific Northwest. The water temperature was about 45 to 50 degrees F (7.2 degrees to 10 degrees C). We were training in dry suits and semi-dry suits. By semi-dry, I mean a wet suit that traps a single layer of water, which the body warms with minimal follow on circulation through the suit. You have probably seen triathlon wet suits that have a slick (versus normal) neoprene surface. A semi-dry wet suit has a similar interior that extends all the way to the wrist, ankle, and neck seals. The advantage is that one layer of water gets into the wet suit or is put there via a hot shower, where it remains. It differs from normal wet suits in that water does not readily circulate through or seep into the suit. Really good ones, like mine, are impregnated with a titanium powder that enhances their insulative properties.

We were conducting very long dives near the limits of the U.S. Navy dive tables. On one dive, after several hours underwater, I approached the hypothermic boundary. I had stopped shivering. [Gordon Giesbrecht noted that when L. Tadeus stopped shivering, he was well past the threshold of mild hypothermia.] At one point during the dive, I actually felt warm, even though my core body temperature was still dropping. Fortunately, the dive ended soon after. When I exited the water, I was very dizzy, suffering from a condition called caloric vertigo—my inner ear on one side was colder than the other, which threw off my balance—so I could barely walk. This appeared to be a neurological deficit consistent with arterial gas embolism (AGE). I was also very lethargic and a little incoherent.

An arterial gas embolism (AGE) can occur during scuba diving. Sometimes simply called gas embolism, it is an obstruction of blood flow caused by gas bubbles (emboli) entering the arterial circulation. Obstruction of the arteries of the brain and heart can lead to death if not promptly relieved. In lay terms: The blood has dissolved gases in it. Dissolved gas can expand and form bubbles with changes in pressure. If those gas bubbles restrict blood flow, especially to the brain, neurological deficits might emerge, such as loss of balance, slurred speech, unilateral coordination, or strength changes.

Diagnosis is difficult, because there are so many things that can cause deficits. For example, if a diver has a balance problem after a dive, it could be because he has caloric vertigo, or he could have AGE (one part of his brain isn't getting oxygen). Determining exactly what is causing the issue can be the difference between a six-hour ride in a small recompression chamber or simple rewarming—ultimately between life and death.

With hypothermia, lethargy and slurred speech are possible. These symptoms are also consistent with AGE. Again, AGE would need to be ruled out.

It took a very long time to rule out a diving-related illness. I didn't have to take a six-hour ride in a recompression chamber, but I was taking neurological exams when what I really wanted to do was sit in a hot tub or curl up in the fetal position and stick my thumb in my mouth in a nice hot shower.

Again, I do not know what my core temp was. I can only speculate that it approached 87 degrees F (30.5 degrees C). But I wasn't any more interested in having my temperature checked rectally than the on-scene doc was in taking my temperature that way. [Gordon Giesbrecht added, "This is precisely why we tell people to measure esophageal temperature. It is easier and thus more likely to be done and more accurate."]

There were distinct portions of the dive I could not recall afterward—I had blank spots in my memory. I do recall feeling very euphoric at the same time I experienced feeling warm. In fact, I recall thinking, Uh-oh, I must be hypothermic . . . cool! I also remember feeling that it was do-or-die, which actually wasn't true. The point is, I was still consciously weighing the length of the rest of the dive against my current perceived condition. In the end, I opted to keep my mouth shut because I was sure the cadre would save me if I got too bad. My symptoms were so apparent to everyone after the dive that the docs had to respond.

The next day, I did not feel hungover. But I remember having a really empty sort of feeling all over. That's the best I can describe it. It took a day or two before that feeling went away.

Hypothermia is something some SEAL trainees experience, especially in the colder months of the year. It usually occurs in Hell Week and during training dives. The instructors recently had a trainee go down right before a chow break early in Hell Week. He was hypoglycemic and cold. It's a bad combination when a person is cold, wet, dehydrated, hasn't slept, and hasn't stopped moving in a couple of days. Rest, hydration, and nutrition are extremely important to high-performance athletes. The trainee's blood oxygen saturation was between 85 and 90 percent. This was a further indicator that he was pretty far gone. His core temp was around 89 degrees F. Below 87 degrees F, most people don't recover.

The trainee was lethargic and incoherent; he stopped shivering and collapsed face-first on the beach. There is a limit to how long a trainee can spend away from his class before he is unable to return. The length of time required for rewarming and feeding this trainee exceeded that limit—trainees cannot return to training until their vital signs are within a certain range.

Trainees exert themselves so much that the instructors have to practically force-feed them all week. The trainees struggle to keep enough calories in them to keep them going. If they don't, hypoglycemia kicks in, and it's only a matter of time before even slight dehydration takes hold.

When this occurs, a lack of circulating fluids means that there is minimal heat generation and minimal heat transfer. The trainee usually spirals downward pretty quickly, but this situation is normal, and on-scene physicians know to deal with it immediately. On rare occasions, a trainee will force himself to power through, and then he does a face-plant.

Years ago, Dr. William Keatinge developed a "thermopill" used by astronauts to measure their core temperatures in space. During my Bering Strait swim, Dr. Keatinge and Dr. Jan Nyboer had me swallow a large metal thermopill so they could monitor my core temperature during the swim in 38-degree F (3.3-degree C) waters. The thermopill transmitted a signal to a receiver on board the escort boat. Unfortunately, the signal dissipated in the salt water; the doctors asked me to roll over on my back so they could hold the receiver near my stomach to get a temperature reading. This was all experimental, and the doctors couldn't obtain good readings, but over the years, the thermopill has been refined. A core temp "pill" is read by an external device to get a core temp periodically without doing anything invasive. The pills are expensive and slightly inaccurate, but well-funded athletes can use it to tell if they need to get warmer/cooler midevent or give support personnel an indication that it is time to stop training and get some medical attention.

Individual Factors

There are individual factors that contribute to a person's ability to acclimate to the cold. Rick Knepper has observed the following:

~ Body fat level is a major factor in preventing hypothermia in the water; however, activity level (the ability to generate heat) is a trade-off dependent on the circumstances. People may react differently to how quickly blood will shut off from the extremities when activity is reduced or stopped.

~ Some swimmers are purists, while others are not. SEAL trainees wear wet suits. If you are going to wear one to prevent hypothermia, Rick explained that you should know how much rubber is in your full or partial wet suit, and swim in it enough times to ensure that you don't get raw spots from rubbing.

~ Seasickness with vomiting can cause a loss of heat from the core and increase the risk of hypothermia.

~ Many first-time hypothermia and hyperthermia incidents probably never would have happened with some sort of evaluation and preparation before a swim.

~ Rick has seen many people recover from both heat exhaustion (not heatstroke) and hypothermia incidents and continue in subsequent training and operations without further incidents. It seems that people become more aware of their capabilities and limitations and make adjustments either to their exposure or their preparation.

~ Many swimmers do not hydrate enough in either hot or cold water, which can lead to problems. Monitor how often you urinate throughout long events.

~ Swimmers who have had a hypothermic incident have been known to increase their body fat and perform well in succeeding events.

~ Whether or not swimmers have had a reaction to heat or cold, they should by all means be very measured in their goals and put controls in place to mitigate and handle any occurrences.

Environmental Factors

Rick pointed out some considerations to make your swims safer:

~ Hot or cold weather conditions may strongly determine if hyperthermia or hypothermia may occur. However, I have seen many cases of hyperthermia that occurred on very cool and overcast days, and cases of hypothermia that occurred on warm, sunny days. Be prepared to recognize both conditions.

~ Weather can change, sometimes significantly. The athlete must be mentally ready to adjust and should have a go and no-go cutoff when temperature or conditions exceed the established thresholds.

~ Paddlers and support crews are vulnerable to heat and cold injuries as well; they need to be ready and dressed accordingly.

~ The sun can be a tremendous factor in heat and sunburn for both swimmer and paddlers. You need to acclimate, get some sun conditioning, and use sun block in ample amounts.

Many swimmers will time their event for the night hours to get calmer water and avoid the sun; this can apply to training swims but does create some safety and support issues when lifeguards are not on duty. Here's another time when a support team of paddlers can provide that safety net.

ICE SWIMMING

For years, people in Russia, Finland, Norway, Denmark, and Sweden have taken saunas, and afterward jumped into ice-cold lakes or rivers and swum for a few meters to invigorate their bodies, and enjoyed the fun. Swimmers around the world participate in these icy dips. On Christmas Day in Dingle, Ireland, Nuala Moore and her lifeguard and open water swimming friends organize a Christmas Day swim for the community. Crowds of people run and shout and jump into the cold water and swim for a few meters as people watch from shore and laugh and encourage them. After the plunge, the swimmers join their friends and warm themselves beside fires and eat bowls of hot soup and mince pies and drink mulled cider, or hot whiskey.

There are communities in the United States and around the world that have annual Polar Bear swims, when people jump into the ocean on New Year's Day to welcome the New Year. It's a great celebration and a lot of fun for the participants and spectators. People are usually aware that they need to get warm immediately after their dip.

There is a new fad emerging in open water swimming described as "ice swimming." Groups of swimmers swim over four hundred meters in water temperatures below 41 degrees F (5 degrees C). They have been encouraging other swimmers to join in.

Recently, three friends who swam the Catalina Channel and are strong swimmers decided to try a mile swim in 41-degree F (5-degree C) water across Lake Arrowhead. Although they'd been training in the ocean, they had not acclimated to the water temperature or to the altitude. One friend said that she jumped into the water and felt pins and needles and, after ten minutes, was very cold. She experienced mild hypothermia, her swimming companion got out after fifteen minutes with moderate hypothermia, and the third swimmer was pulled out after twenty minutes, taken to the emergency room with severe hypothermia, and spent a day in the hospital.

Ice swimming can be dangerous even if a swim is only four hundred meters. It should never been done as a lark. It has taken me over thirty years to swim in very cold water, and when I do a very cold swim, I spend a great deal of time acclimating and have lifeguard and medical support alongside me on my swim.

AFTER-DROP

After most cool- or cold-water swims, swimmers will have an after-drop, meaning that once they're out of the water, increased blood flow to the colder limbs cools the blood, which then returns to cool the heart further. Most swimmers will feel chilled after a cold swim, and some will shiver; this is often a result of after-drop and a colder brain temperature. Though shivering is the body's protective mechanism to create heat, and it helps the body rewarm, most swimmers do not enjoy the after-drop or the intense shivering.

After my two-hour-and-six-minute swim across the Bering Strait in water temperatures that ranged from 38 to 42 degrees F (3.3 to 5.5 degrees C), I experienced after-drop. The Russian physician, Dr. Rita Zacharova, was extremely well versed in treatment for hypothermia. She prepared a rewarming tent, a shelter that was far warmer than the icy Siberian beach on Big Diomede Island.

Dr. Zacharova had me remove my wet swimsuit, dry off, and climb into a sleeping bag. She placed a hot-water bottle on my forearm to make sure it wasn't too hot, and then she applied bottles on either side of my neck, under each arm, and in my groin. The heat from the bottles warmed the blood in large arteries near the skin surface; this warmed blood circulated through my body and warmed my core effectively; and I shivered moderately, which was my body's way of generating heat. Within an hour, my core temperature had risen to 102 degrees F (38.8 degrees C), well above my normal 97.6 F (36.4 degrees C).

After-drop is not something any swimmer wants to undergo. I've learned from experience and from the United States Air Force, which conducts cold survival training in Greenland and Antarctica, to put on warm, dry clothes after a swim, get into a warm environment, drink warm fluids, eat food for rewarming, and (only if you know that you are not significantly hypothermic) keep moving to generate heat. If my skin is very cold, what works for me is to take a cool shower and gradually increase the water temperature until it is hot, then put on warm clothes and drink warm fluids and eat something to give my body fuel.

Chapter 8

Sinuses and Ears

For years, I taught children and adults how to swim. Often parents told me they were concerned that their children would develop ear or sinus infections. Once that occurred, the children seemed to be more susceptible to other infections.

Last summer, a friend traveled with his young family to Finland for vacation. His son swam in a beautiful clear freshwater lake. A few days after the swim, the son developed an ear infection. When the Finnish doctor looked at his ears, he said, "In all the years I've treated patients, I've never seen a child with algae growing out of his ears." The doctor treated the infection and the child was fine, but his father told me that his son always gets ear infections now. Earplugs might have helped.

PREVENTION OF INFECTIONS

Some swimmers use a type of silicone earplug that shapes itself to ears like wax or putty, prevents most water from getting into the ear canal, and helps to prevent ear infections.

Other swimmers use plastic earplugs—make sure they fit snugly in your ears. Most of the swimsuit manufacturers and swim and surf shops carry a variety of earplugs.

The only problem with earplugs is that when you put them in your ears, you reduce your ability to hear what's going on around you. You might not hear an approaching boater, Jet Skier, or kite surfer. When I needed to wear earplugs, I made sure to be even more observant while I was swimming to compensate for not being to hear as well. When I swam in Antarctica, I was not sure how the 32-degree temperature would affect my ears and whether exposure would injure my ears. I tried using plastic earplugs, but they were uncomfortable. When I was visiting William Poe, my dentist, I mentioned that I was trying to find a way to protect my ears. He said that his son was always getting ear infections, so he custom-made a pair for him using dental material. He offered to do the same for me. He squeezed the dental material in my ears and let the material form to my ear canals. When he removed them, he labeled them "right" and "left" so I would be able to tell them apart.

They kept my ear canals completely dry and, unlike some hard plastic earplugs, did not irritate the ear canals when I pulled them out. The earplugs reduced my hearing somewhat, but my support boats were all within twenty feet of me, and I could hear the crew clearly.

The SEALs spend a lot of time conducting dive training, and it is critical for them to have clear sinuses and ears so they don't rupture their eardrums or get a blocked sinus. They have figured out that the causes of the sinus and ear infections determine how they treat the infections. For example, if a person has adult-onset allergies and routinely has sinus infections, there are preventative meds, such as Allegra and nose sprays, that keep the infections at bay. Some SEALs deal with infections as they happen. They have also found that if a person is otherwise healthy, simple hygiene should do the trick. Q-tips do wonders for the ears. The SEALs have seen many trainees get "squeezes" (the inability to equalize pressure between two air spaces) due to dirty ears. A squeeze can happen in the inner ears (and can result in perforation of the tympanic membrane—a "perf," as they call it).

A perf can happen while ascending (a reverse squeeze) or descending. This is much more problematic when the trainee needs to get to the surface. If it happens going down, they can always stop and go back up. Stopping to go back down isn't always an option, especially when they don't have enough air.

To keep the sinuses free of muck, a squirt of saline solution in the nose will work (saline doesn't burn too much). The SEALs avoid Afrin because the body builds a tolerance to it. Eventually, the sinuses cannot do their job without the Afrin.

Chapter 9

Ocean Hazards

FOG

Swimming in fog can be very risky. It is possible to get lost right offshore and out in the middle of the channel. Years ago, Jim Murray, an amazing sportswriter for the *Los Angeles Times*, recounted his story about swimming off the shore of Boston with his brother. They were preteens and had decided to go for a swim. Jim was nearsighted and didn't have goggles with corrective lenses. They were swimming just offshore when the fog swept in. Jim lost sight of his brother. He shouted his name but heard nothing. Jim started to get scared. The fog was swirling around him and closing in.

He wanted to swim to shore, but he couldn't tell which way to go. He tried turning around and swimming toward where he thought the shore would be, but after swimming for some time, he didn't find shore. He tried swimming in another direction and shouted his brother's name again, but all he heard was the loud moan of the foghorn. He was cold and getting colder and could feel the fear in him rising to panic. He wondered if he was going to die. He talked himself into swimming again. He tried moving in a different direction, and suddenly, a white buoy loomed in front of him. He found a chain and clung to it for hours and felt the cold moving into his body and chilling him to the bone.

When the fog finally lifted, he swam in to shore and found his brother, who had been lost in the fog onshore, about a half mile down the beach from where they had left their towels. It took Jim hours to warm up, and he never quite got over the experience.

Even though I had an experienced crew, I got lost at night in the middle of the Catalina Channel. These are the things I do to avoid being lost in the fog:

~ Don't get in the water if the fog is moving in.
~ Wear a GPS or compass wristwatch and know how to use it.
~ Swim just outside the wave break so that if the fog moves in, you can hear the surf and turn in to shore.
~ Wear a bright-colored swim cap.
~ If possible, swim beside support vessels with good illumination.

I asked L. Tadeus what the SEALs do if they get caught in the fog and how they implement safety measures to prevent being lost. He said, "If we are conducting a training swim with trainees and I have doubts about my ability to keep them safe, we reschedule the swim. If I am swimming and fog rolls in, I always have an analog compass on my watch. Some watches have a compass function built in. By knowing the long shore bearing, I can simply swim at ninety degrees to it and find my way back to shore—mission planning [discussed in Chapter 12]. If I am near surf, I just listen for it and swim to it. GPS is an awesome tool, but electronics and seawater have a long history of not working well together. Usually, GPS fails right when you need it. We have a mantra in the SEAL teams: "Two is one, one is none." Always have a redundant method for everything, including navigation. The goal is to carefully think it through—time-critical risk management."

SHIPS, BOATS, JET SKIS, SAILOR BOATS, WINDSURFERS, KITE SURFERS, AND SURFERS

Never assume that people operating watercrafts see you. You must always be watching and aware and make sure you get out of their way. Many people who are operating watercrafts are not looking for swimmers, or they are distracted.

Recently, a friend contacted me to say that she'd heard about a new device that a swimmer could wear to listen to music. She wanted to know if the sounds emitted by the device might attract sharks. My response was: Don't worry about the sharks; worry about the boaters, windsurfers, and anyone else on the water. If you are listening to music, you may not be able to hear the engine sounds of a small boat and most will not hear a windsurfer sailing by. It would be bad to get a skeg in the head. My friend said that she was planning to swim in an area that was designated for swimmers with buoys, and I said that while boaters are told they cannot operate in swimming areas, they sometimes stray, and if you are wearing head-phones, you may not hear the boater.

If you want to wear a headset and listen to music, do it in a swimming pool. Most people who are swimming in the open water want to hear what's happening around them and enjoy being out there.

PART TWO

Beginning and Intermediate Swimmers

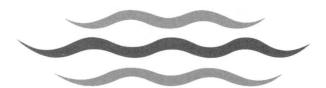

Chapter 10

Training Swims

Training swims are just that—they give you the chance to test your ability, monitor your improvement, try different foods and liquids before big swims and competitions. Training swims will help you find what works best for you and how frequently you need to feed and in what sequence to eat and drink. They give you the opportunity to test yourself before big swims or competitions. Whether short or long, these swims need to be planned in detail like a mission.

L. Tadeus noted that mission planning and progressive training plans are equally important. He said, "Besides mission planning, probably the most important risk-management tool we use is a progressive training plan. Obviously, you do not jump into the water and knock out a ten-mile swim on your first day. You build intensity, whether that is through added duration, added distance, added speed, or added environmental challenges."

In open water training sessions, pool swimmers and triathletes work on pace, speed, intensity, endurance, and stroke just like they would in the swimming pool. In the open water, you will need to be able to sprint and have endurance. The sprinting ability helps you move through currents and tidal changes, and the endurance training enables you to swim long distances without having to rest.

When I transitioned from the swimming pool to the ocean, Ron Blackledge, the Seal Beach swim coach who let me train with his team, applied workouts from the swimming pool in the ocean. He had us work on pace, speed, intensity, endurance, and stroke. In the swimming pool, we would swim ten times one hundred yards freestyle on a pace of one minute and thirty seconds. We would descend each one hundred, or swim each one faster than the previous swim. In the ocean, we would swim ten miles (sixteen kilometers), each mile on a twenty-one-minute interval and faster than the previous mile.

If I hadn't trained for three years with Don Gambril, the four-time Olympic swimming coach, and Ben Muritt, the Harvard University swim coach, for four years during summer vacation, and club coaches in the winter, I would not have been able to jump into the ocean and swim with the Seal Beach team. Even though I had a great basis, in my first week, Coach Blackledge had me swim half to three-quarters the distance, because ocean swimming requires far more energy than pool swimming, and he wanted me to succeed and be able to build on my success. If I'd been unable to complete the workout, I might have been discouraged, and it would have taken more energy and focus to overcome that.

Once Coach Blackledge saw that I could complete the workouts and I wasn't getting overly tired or injured, he allowed me to swim the entire workout. When I decided to swim across the English Channel, Coach Gambril agreed to coach me and increased the intensity and varied the distances. I swam hard through the workouts, and I got stronger, but I also took time to recover so I could build on what I was doing, swim longer with more intensity, and get even stronger.

The SEALs carefully plan their workouts like missions,

even if they are swimming only a mile or two. Make sure that every time you go into the water, you plan, mitigate risk, swim where there are lifeguards, and swim with a buddy or buddies.

TRAINING SAFELY

One of the key concepts Rick Knepper has learned during his years as an instructor and swimmer is that even the best swimmers in the world can have serious problems during routine workouts. Based on these experiences, he recommends:

~ Swim with a swimming buddy who knows your capabilities and can identify if something is going wrong.
~ If you run into trouble in the open water before lifeguards come on duty, get the attention of people onshore and have them call 911 for help. Be relentless. Continue to shout and signal for help until it is rendered.
~ Know what you are capable of doing and how much help you can render.

From years of experience, Rick has seen all sorts of swimmers, all levels of accomplishment, and various factors that set people up for problems. These are things he thinks you need to keep in mind when you're swimming in the open water:

~ The person in trouble is usually the last one to recognize that anything is wrong.
~ Experience in various conditions gives a positive edge but does not guarantee anything.
~ Each season and workout are different; people get older, fitness levels change with life, and constant reas-

sessment of goals and milestones is necessary, even within the season.

~ People are at risk when attempting an event distance in conditions that are too far beyond what they have previously done; swimmers need to expand or extend personal capabilities in a measured way to be aware of their current limits and abilities.

~ Acclimation is a huge factor. You need to get into the water enough times to adapt to the conditions; the mind acclimates as well as the body.

~ When you are training in very cold or hot water, take some recovery time to prevent overtraining.

~ Mental conditioning is important: You need to work on goal segmenting, arousal control, visualization, and positive self-talk.

~ Symptoms of hypothermia and hyperthermia may vary among people. Some swimmers may naturally slow down during a swim; others, however, may experience a sharp breakdown in stroke count, a sign that something is wrong.

~ Athletes, especially the serious ones, are mentally tough and will push through extreme zones. A team leader needs to know the swimmer and make the right call on whether to stop or encourage the swimmer.

~ People have different tolerances to heat and cold dependent upon many genetic and fitness factors. Rick has seen people shivering uncontrollably and mentally out of it with a core temperature of 96 degrees F (35.5 degrees C), while other swimmers with core temperatures between 88 and 92 degrees F (31.1 and 33.3 degrees C) are talking normally and shaking moderately despite being in serious danger.

~ Athletes can bring on a problem before an event, such as through improper training. It's better to be undertrained and rested than to be overtrained and tired.

~ One of the worst things you can do as a swimmer is to try a new food or fluid before a swim. The food or fluid might make you sick and cause you to abort the swim. Stick to your feeding plans. Swim like you trained.

~ Improper taper: Make sure to reduce your training gradually, and get enough rest before your big swim.

TRAINING FOR A SHORT OPEN WATER SWIM

The most important things when you start swimming in the open water are: Identify your current swimming level, figure out what your goals are, and draft a progressive training plan that will help you reach your goal. Will you be training for a short, medium, or long triathlon or open water swim? Can you set goals that will help you gradually build strength, speed, and endurance? Figuring out your swimming level, goals, and plan to achieve your goals is easier if you have a coach who can give you feedback and guidance.

I'm defining a short swim as between one mile (1.6 kilometers) and three miles (4.8 kilometers), because there are many age groups, triathletes, and masters swimmers who routinely complete these distances during pool workouts. A medium distance suitable for intermediate and advanced swimmers would be four to ten miles (6.4 to 16 kilometers), and a long distance for advanced swimmers would be anything over ten miles (16 kilometers).

When you are considering the length of the swim, remember that you most likely will not swim a straight line from one point to another, and the distance will be a little or perhaps a lot longer than what was defined. You need to consider the environmental factors that will influence the distance of your swim.

When you are entering the open water, you may experience a sense of excitement at being in water that is alive and filled with life. You may feel a sense of freedom that you no longer have to swim back and forth in a lane, and flip-turn off cement walls, and follow a black line on the bottom of the pool. You may enjoy breathing fresh air and love being able to swim from one place to another.

There are some swimmers, runners, and triathletes who feel overwhelmed when they get in the water. The open water seems ominous. They are afraid. They can't hang on pool walls and lane lines. They can't see the bottom and can't follow the black line to help them stay on course. They have to allow themselves time to become comfortable in the water. They need to swim with a confident and helpful swimming buddy.

Your first open water swims should be brief—between ten to twenty minutes long and a distance of a half mile. If you have difficulty telling the distance in the open water, figure out how many strokes it takes you to swim one hundred yards in a pool and use the stroke count to estimate the distance you are swimming in the open water.

Gradually get into the water with your swimming buddy, and enjoy the new sensations of being in the open water. Talk about what you are seeing, feeling, experiencing. It should be a lot of fun. A lot of swimmers and triathletes use this time to crack jokes, review the way they plan to swim, and relish the feeling of leaving land and entering the water and being lifted off their feet.

Try swimming alongside the buoy to help you swim in a straight line. When you breathe, look around at the water, the waves, and the people walking alongshore. Listen to what's going on around you.

Take your time to stretch out your arms and slip into your pace. If you are swimming in the ocean, notice how much more buoyant you are in the salt water, and if you are swimming in fresh water, feel the water's effervescence. You may notice that the salt water feels denser than pool water, and fresh water tastes sweeter. You may notice on a summer's day how the sun warms the trees, grass, and flowers, and how you can detect the direction of the wind by the scent in the air, long before you see ripples on the water.

As you become more familiar with your new "pool," you will see more of what's happening around you. You may notice the changing sky and sea. You may see small black water bugs with their legs splayed, skimming the surface of a lake. You may have sunfish pop from below and nibble on your toes. You may find yourself drawn into the magic of exploration, punctuated with moments of discovery. Savor these experiences with friends after your swims are completed.

In your next workout, add two to five minutes or one hundred to two hundred meters. Take time to feel the water and the way the currents push and pull you. You may have to work harder to get through a current, or you may swim across a glassy sea that is calmer than the swimming pool.

People have different training backgrounds, schedules, and time that they can dedicate to open water swimming. Training is most effective if you work out daily and gradually add time and distance to your swims. By training daily, you will become stronger, more relaxed in the water, able to acclimate to the water temperatures, and make steady progress.

Add time and distance to your swims in five- to ten-minute increments. If you are not able to get into the open water daily, your conditioning may take longer than that of someone who works out every day in the open water. Whether you are able to train every day or only a couple of times a week, the key to swimming a mile or more is to spend time in the water, adding distance incrementally so you build strength and remain injury free.

Continue adding time and distance to swims until you reach your mile goal. If you need to take shorter swims because of fatigue or limited time, do it. Give yourself time to recover. Everyone conditions differently. Your goal is to swim a mile comfortably. Take time to watch the clouds or a dragonfly and sip water.

If you're training for a mile swim or a two- or three-mile swim, the distance you'll swim will be farther, so you may want to add at least half a mile (one-eighth of a kilometer) to your training distance to compensate for the current. It is always better to be overprepared than underprepared. Once you reach the mile goal, you can start working on your speed, which is as important as distance. You need to be able to pick up your pace and sprint to get through currents. Currents can play a huge role in a swim, and if you cannot sprint when you need to, you may not be able to complete your race.

You can work on developing your speed by swimming faster with your buddy. Sprint for two hundred strokes or two hundred yards (182.9 meters), then swim one hundred yards (91.4 meters) at a moderate pace. Alternate this pace and speed work for the entire mile; or you can warm up in the first half mile, stretching out and working on your stroke, then alternate between sprint and pace on the second half mile. The key is to sprint and give yourself time to recover. Be creative with your workouts. If you're swimming a mile, you can break down the distance into quarter miles (four hundred meters) and swim each quarter mile faster than the last so that your body learns how to become stronger as you work longer.

You can also break the mile down into one-hundred-stroke sections. Swim one hundred strokes fast; one hundred strokes moderate; and one hundred strokes in which you focus on your stroke. Then build back up to swimming one hundred strokes moderately and then one hundred strokes fast. The more you train, the more you familiarize yourself with the open water, the more comfortable you'll be, and the more able you'll be to focus on your swimming, enjoy the open water, and see yourself progress. There are triathletes who are in incredible shape for running and cycling, but they are concerned about their open water swims. I often hear triathletes say, "If I can just get through the swimming, I'll be okay." Most triathletes work hard to prepare for the swimming and do great, but some look at the swimming as a relatively short distance and don't take the time to prepare. This is unfortunate, because swimming can be more dangerous than riding a bike or running. If a triathlete gets tired when riding a bike or running, he or she can stop, but in the open water, there is no place to rest. The more prepared they are for the open water swimming, the more relaxed they will be, and then they'll be able to use their energy for the next two parts of the race. Once you have completed your one-mile distance and feel comfortable in the water, you can gradually increase your distances and continue to work on pace, speed, stroke, and navigation.

Some Ideas for a Three-Mile (4.8-Kilometer) Swim

WORKOUT 1

1. Swim freestyle. Break the three miles (4.8 kilometers) into six half-mile swims (or six 0.8-kilometer swims). Swim a half mile at pace and a half mile at a sprint.

2. Swim another half mile at a slightly faster pace and the second half mile faster than your first sprint.

3. Swim the third mile pace faster than your second, and sprint the last half mile faster than your previous sprint.

4. Give yourself thirty seconds to a minute rest between each mile (1.6-kilometer) swim. Get your times during your workouts, record them, and monitor your progress.

WORKOUT 2

1. Break the three miles (4.8 kilometers) into one-mile (1.6-kilometer) segments. Warm up by swimming the first mile freestyle at pace.

2. Break the second mile into four one-hundred-meter segments. Swim each four hundred meters faster than the previous four hundred.

3. For the last mile, swim two hundred strokes at pace, two hundred sprint, three hundred pace, three hundred sprint, four hundred pace, four hundred sprint, three hundred pace, three hundred sprint, two hundred pace, two hundred sprint, one hundred pace, one hundred sprint. Continue through this drill until you complete the third mile.

Swimming head-up in the open water can become a bad habit, but it is important that you can see what's going on around you, navigate, and be more visible if watercrafts stray into your swimming area.

Because swimming head-up puts more stress on your shoulders, be sure that you warm up with your normal freestyle stroke for a half mile (0.8 kilometers), then alternate the next half mile between swimming head-up for one hundred strokes and head-down for four hundred. Break the second mile (1.6 kilometers) into two half-mile swims. In the first half mile, alternate between two hundred strokes butterfly and backstroke; in the second half mile, alternate between two hundred strokes breaststroke and freestyle. For the last mile, swim the first half mile freestyle and concentrate on your stroke. Focus on your catch, pull, and recovery. For the last half mile, swim freestyle, and build your speed from moderate to fast. Finish with a sprint. Usually, by the end of an open water or triathlon race, the wind or current has picked up, and if you have trained to swim stronger at the end of your workout, you can replicate it at the end of your race.

It would be unfair for me to write a series of workouts and tell you that if you follow this manual, you will reach your goals. Reading a book will help you prepare and give you a sense of what to do, but you cannot become an open water swimmer or triathlete by reading a manual, just like you can't become a SEAL by reading a manual. You have to put in the time, distance, and training to reach your goals.

Last year, a friend of mine signed up for her first short triathlon. The distance of her swim was four hundred meters in a fifty-meter pool. She hadn't swum four hundred meters before, but she thought that if she signed up for the triathlon, it would give her the motivation to learn. She had surfed before but did not know how to swim and breathe correctly. She contacted me and asked if I'd help her. After five lessons, she had the basics and said she would work out, but she dreaded it and did not do much training. I went to watch her at the triathlon. She had to hang on to the lane lines and the wall to catch her breath, and she barely made the four hundred meters, but she was really proud of herself. She said she intended to do more triathlons, and I said they would be a lot easier if she put in more time in the water.

Recently, during a workout at the gym, she told me she had signed up for a triathlon and would be swimming a mile in a lake. I asked if she had been swimming, and she said, "Yes, a little," and I asked if she was swimming more than when she'd trained for the four hundred meters in the pool. She said no. I couldn't believe that she was planning to swim four times the distance of her first swim without any real training. I was concerned that she might not make it. Her response was if she ran into trouble, there were people on kayaks who could help her. I just couldn't understand this mentality. She was doing less than minimal to prepare. Not only did that set her up for failure, it was also danger-ous. In a triathlon, during the run, you can walk; during the cycling, you can slow down; but during the swimming, you have to be strong, especially when you are with a lot of other swimmers who are heading for the same buoy and there is a high possibility of unintentionally knocking into another swimmer or being swum over. Although there is kayak and boat support, there are so many swimmers in the water that the support people may not immediately see you. It is not wise to be unprepared for open water swims.

Raylene Movius, a friend who competes in outrigger canoe and dragon boat races and is a world champion in both, says that "we train like we race, and we race like we train." It is the same with open water swimming, and you will discover that as you get better, you'll enjoy being out in the open water more, feeling the natural rhythms of the water and wind, and listening to the calls of seabirds or laughter of friends.

TRAINING FOR A MODERATE OR LONG OPEN WATER SWIM

When you are training for a moderate or long open water swim, your time commitment is considerably longer. You will experience more current and tidal changes and weather than you would on a short swim. It is fun to see what you are capable of achieving. For many open water swimmers and triathletes, the open water swims become meditative, a chance to think about challenges in their lives and to find solutions. During college, I spent a lot of time memorizing information or thinking about history or English papers I would write when I climbed out of the ocean.

The key to swimming the moderate and long swims is to continue to build progressively on your training and to add in rest and recovery time and work with a coach.

When I started open water swimming, I was training between five and ten miles (eight and sixteen kilometers) per day for the San Pedro Channel (Catalina) and the

English Channel. My workouts were between two to four hours a day, and they varied in distance and intensity each day. For a while, Dave, my older brother, coached me and swam with me, since he was training for the English Channel while I was training to swim the Catalina Channel. We varied our workout sites so that we could experience different conditions.

When we swam off Long Beach, California, we usually swam from the Long Beach pier to the jetty near 62nd Place and back. The distance was five miles (eight kilometers), and we always encountered strong currents as we neared 62nd Place. Sometimes we did two trips and covered ten miles (sixteen kilometers). We also swam off Seal Beach and broke our swims into half-mile segments when we swam from the Seal Beach Pier to the northern jetty and back, a mile round-trip. We worked on our pace because we had a set mile course and kept track of our times each day. The currents did not vary much from day to day, and we were able to easily monitor our progress. We also swam along Sunset Beach, where there was a lot more surf and stronger currents. Sometimes we would swim near the northern jetty at Surfside and swim in place for half an hour because the current was so strong. At Huntington Beach, the surf was typically three to eight feet (0.9 to 2.4 meters), and the current sometimes was so strong that when we tried to swim forward, we were pushed backward for the entire workout. What we learned was to keep working, keep going, and keep trying to swim faster than the current. There were times when we had the current at our backs, and we'd fly across the water at double our speed. It was so much fun, especially after swimming into a current and seeing little or no progress.

It will be a challenge to figure out what you need to do to train for a moderate to long open water swim. It is important to be totally prepared, though it is equally important to make sure that you don't overtrain. There was one coach I swam with, after Don Gambril, who also coached Olympic swimmers. This coach believed that if you were a distance swimmer, you needed to do excessive distances in the pool, up to ten miles a day, and when he coached me, he felt that I needed to swim six hours or roughly fifteen miles (24.1 kilometers) a day. After two weeks of these workouts, I was too tired to sleep, didn't want to eat, and lost twenty pounds (nine kilograms) and my love of swimming. All of this contributed to failure on my attempt to swim the Catalina Channel and break the records, but I took two weeks off from swimming, went back to doing the workouts that Dave and I created, which were no longer than ten miles a day, and a few weeks later, I achieved my goal.

The key is to listen to your body and be honest with yourself, to know when you can push yourself and when you need to rest.

Here are a few workouts for moderate and long swims, to give you some ideas. Your level of conditioning and experience may differ from someone else's, so you need to develop workouts specifically for yourself—if you can, with a coach or other open water swimmers who will give you the daily input you need to reach your goals.

Some Ideas for a Five-Mile (Eight-Kilometer) Swim

WORKOUT 1

1. Warm up for the first mile (0.8 kilometers) and focus on your stroke.

2. Swim two miles (3.2 kilometers) and break them into eight four-hundred-meter swims/quarter-mile segments. Alternate between sprinting four hundred meters and swimming at moderate pace.

3. Swim two miles at your pace.

WORKOUT 2

1. Swim a one-mile (0.8-kilometer) warm-up.

2. Swim one mile: two hundred strokes fast, two hundred strokes moderate, three hundred strokes fast, three hundred strokes moderate, four hundred strokes fast, four hundred strokes moderate. Stretch out for four hundred strokes and repeat until you complete the mile (1.6-kilometer) swim.

3. Swim three miles (4.8 kilometers) at your pace, trying to make each mile as close in time as you can.

As a way to develop your sense of pace, have a friend walk the beach while you swim at the same pace as the person walking. This becomes challenging when you are swimming against a current, but you want to develop a way to feel the speed of the current. When you are on a channel swim or a swim between islands or across a bay, you may not be able to see the shore to gauge your speed, so you need to be able to judge the speed of the current and adjust your effort when you are swimming with or against it.

When you are swimming long distances, it is really important to work on your pace and your endurance, and your training should reflect that.

Suggestions for a Ten-Mile (Sixteen-Kilometer) Swim

WORKOUT 1

1. Swim five miles (eight kilometers) broken into two segments. Swim the first two and a half miles (four kilometers) at your pace. Swim the second two-and-a-

half-mile segment faster than your pace. Focus on the entry (or catch) part of your stroke.

2. On a long open water swim, you will experience the effects of currents and tides for a longer time period. You will need to sustain your sprinting capability until you can break through the tide or current. Swim at sprint speed for two and a half miles so you have completed seven and a half miles.

3. For the remaining two and a half miles, swim each half mile (0.8 kilometers) faster than the previous. Make sure to stretch out and loosen up for at least four hundred meters.

WORKOUT 2

1 mile = 1.6 kilometers

1. Swim a one-mile warm-up.

2. Swim your second mile at a moderate pace.

3. Swim your third mile as a sprint.

4. Swim your fourth mile at a moderate pace.

5. Swim your fifth mile fast.

6. During your sixth mile, stretch out and focus on your stroke.

7. During your seventh mile, alternate five hundred strokes freestyle with five hundred strokes backstroke.

8. During your eighth mile, alternate five hundred strokes butterfly with five hundred strokes breaststroke.

9. Swim your ninth mile as a sprint.

10. Swim your tenth mile at pace.

Suggestion for a Fifteen-Mile Swim

You will need a competent kayaker on this swim for safety and navigation and so you can hydrate and eat. Pick out a course alongshore that will allow you to swim 7.5 miles (12 kilometers) with a turnaround point. Look carefully at the map and note the distances, for example, between the pier and a cove, between a cove and a peninsula, or between a peninsula and a sandy beach. Use these points to create your workout: Warm up by swimming from the pier to the cove; work on your pace by swimming from the cove to the peninsula; sprint from the peninsula to the sandy beach. These workouts are really fun, and you get to create them as you are doing them.

You may also want to swim fifteen miles (24.1 kilometers) from one point to another. Years ago, Louise Comar—a friend who was training to swim the Catalina Channel—and I swam just outside the wave break from the Malibu Pier to the Santa Monica Pier. It was a fifteen-mile (24.1-kilometer) swim, and while it was tough, and we got tired off and on during the swim, we had fun swimming from one point to another, from a cluster of homes to a stand of palm trees at our pace, or from an outcropping of boulders around a cove to the Hearst Museum at sprint speed.

We worked hard when we swam into a current and tried to maintain our pace; we stretched out our strokes and moved closer to the water's surface and let the sun warm our backs. This swim gave Louise the confidence to continue training and complete the Catalina Channel swim.

If you plan to swim across a channel, these long swims with kayak, Zodiac, or boat support will help you prepare. They give you a chance to mentally and physically understand what it's like to swim for a long distance, and they will give you a chance to work with some of your crew so that they know what kind of support you need and how you are doing during your swim.

The crew will also be able to observe you during your training and get to know you better. They will be able to see if your stroke looks strong, if you're pulling or slipping water. They'll be able to time your stroke rate and see if you're swimming on pace. They will be able to tell if you're working hard or struggling and should be able to tell if you are injured or showing symptoms of hypothermia or hyperthermia.

These swims are training swims, and you always want to complete them if you can, but if the weather conditions suddenly deteriorate, or you are not feeling well, or things are going wrong, it is better to stop the swim and recover and come back and complete it another day. The last thing you want to do is injure yourself and then be out of the water longer than if you'd climbed out. Longer swims are great indicators of how well you've trained. You can time each swim and repeat the courses to see your progress. Sometimes you will see a big increase in speed, and sometimes (say, if water conditions are rough) you will see a slower speed, but every time you swim in the open water, you will gather new experiences that will help you on longer swims.

Chapter 11

Selection for Support and Swim

SKILLS REQUIRED FOR A KAYAKER

Most long open water swims—especially channel swims—require an escort boat or multiple escort boats, depending on the channel and the number of swimmers. Kayakers are a fantastic complement to the escort boats. They are able to make sure a swimmer is doing okay and can maneuver closer than an escort boat.

To prepare for an open water swim, a kayaker must be able to kayak through surf, to keep the swimmer on a straight course, and in case of emergency, to respond and get a lifesaving device secured around a swimmer or help her hang on to the kayak until the escort boat can provide additional assistance.

A kayaker must be able to direct a swimmer around kelp, rocks, and underwater obstructions. Let the kayaker know what is needed to help you on your swim so you'll know if he is capable of fulfilling your requirements.

KAYAKER SELECTION

Here is the method the SEALs use to select a qualified kayaker:

~ Publish in a public place that you are seeking help and have people send in applications with a drop-dead date planned backward from your race/open water swim.
~ Mandate that applicants furnish evidence of experience, and mandate references (training attended, races supported, lives saved).
~ Toss all the iffy applications in the trash, along with all the ones that arrive late.
~ Set up interviews with the top three candidates after calling their references and asking specific questions about skill levels.
~ Make applicants demonstrate their competence by setting up a kayak obstacle course, including pulling you from the water.

KAYAKER COMPETENCY

The SEALs generate a short critical task list (CTL) to demonstrate a kayaker's competency. The first indicator is if she shows up with the necessary equipment: life jacket, Warmies, waterproof bags, paddle, sunscreen, food, water, seat, aqua socks or water shoes and gloves, rescue buoy, flashlight, extra glow sticks, whistle, and extra batteries.

A qualified kayaker needs to know:

~ The rules (no touching the swimmer, how to pass food and drink)
~ How to operate a GPS
~ How to operate a radio/phone/walkie-talkie

~ How to set up the kayak
~ How to launch the kayak
~ How to get through surf—not in Lake Pacific surf but in Morro Bay surf
~ How to paddle for a long distance, specific to the needs of the swim
~ Demonstrate swimmer tow
~ Demonstrate swimmer rescue
~ How to right the kayak and save herself
~ Go over various mishap scenarios

SWIMMING ROUTE

It is best to swim with people who know a swimming area and to check in with lifeguards and ask questions about the water conditions on that specific day. The SEALs and I created the following list of things you need to consider before you swim in the open water:

1. Route

    Before swimming in any waterway, you need to identify and weigh the dangers:

    ~ Where are the shipping lanes? Will you be staying clear of the ships?
    ~ Where are the surf zones? Is the tide coming in or going out?
    ~ Are there shallow obstacles, such as pier pilings, that you can swim into?
    ~ Are there dynamic fishing nets and fishing lines that you can get tangled in?
    ~ Are there submerged rocks that you can swim into?
    ~ What are the risks in dangerous areas, and what can you do before the swim to mitigate the risks?

2. Environmental Factors

   ~ What is the weather on the day you plan to swim?
   ~ What is the water quality?
   ~ What is the water temperature?
   ~ Have you spoken with local authorities about the swimming area?
   ~ Is there a local jellyfish bloom?
   ~ Are there sea snakes or dangerous animals?

3. Emergency Action Plan

   ~ Do you know what to do if something happens to your swimming buddy (or buddies) during the swim?
   ~ Do you know how to contact lifeguards?
   ~ Do you have a cell phone and the numbers for local emergency responders?
   ~ Do you have coast guard contact numbers?
   ~ Do you know how to provide transport to the hospital?

4. What Are the Minimum Requirements for the Support Pilot/Boat?

   ~ What are the qualifications of the pilot?
   ~ Does he have certificates?
   ~ Has the boat been maintained?
   ~ What are the maintenance records on the motors, and is there a spare motor?
   ~ What is the maintenance record on the boat—has it been maintained periodically?
   ~ Has it been inspected by the coast guard?
   ~ What kind of medical training has the pilot had?
   ~ What type of supplies does the captain have on the boat?

~ Are there life jackets, survival suits, life rafts?

~ Do you have communication equipment: cell phone, radio, whistle, smoke, flare gun?

~ What is the medical equipment on board?

~ What type of maintenance has been done on the motors, and how periodically? Is there a spare?

~ Is the pilot willing to do swim support rehearsals and emergency rehearsals?

~ What is the go/no-go plan?

~ What is the threshold for the swimmer?

~ What is the threshold for the boat/kayak/Jet Ski? Can it be maneuvered in and out of surf or is it too high?

PART THREE

Intermediate
and
Advanced Swimmers

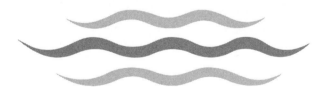

Chapter 12

Open Water Swims Outside the Buoys with Boat Support

These guidelines are helpful in planning an open water swim that goes beyond the swimming buoys and requires an escort boat and kayaks. Because conditions are changing constantly, it is important to use this information just as a guideline, to be aware of what's happening in the water throughout the swim, and to adjust to ensure the safety of the swimmer, crew, and boat. It is critical to the success of a swim to have the pilot and crew act as professionally as possible. These guidelines were developed with the invaluable recommendations of the U.S. Navy SEAL officer/instructor L. Tadeus.

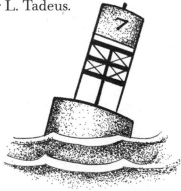

INFORMATION GATHERING/RESEARCH

There is no "one size fits all" when it comes to swimming and surface support—unless you are funded for maximal support and have a small navy following you on every swim. Swimmers need to take things like this into account when they plan for a swim. The surface support required in great weather is minimal, and the surface support required in bad weather is maximal. It will take more people on the boat to help when the waves are big and the rain is coming down like sheets of lead.

The SEAL stressed:

~ Gather as much information as possible about the area where you intend to swim.
~ What are the prevailing meteorological and oceanographic conditions during the time of year when you plan to swim?
~ What are the go/no-go criteria for the swim (the worst possible conditions you would want to swim in)? Consider your ability and the crew's and the support boats'. Swimmers, crews, and boats will have different thresholds.
~ Know what water temperature to expect, and study the currents, winds, and waves.
~ Research the dangerous marine life in the water and treatments for run-ins.
~ You can't beat local knowledge of an area. Talk to someone who is familiar with those waters.
~ As the time of the swim draws near, consult the most specific and up-to-date weather forecasts.
~ Visit the location before the swim. It helps to see the starting point and finish in advance, although on many swims, you won't know where you will finish until you get there.
~ Conduct short recreational swims in that location—you could learn something while at play.

SELECTING SUPPORT CREW

~ How much support do you need?
~ What is the required team makeup?
~ What individual qualifications are required?
~ What training is required for each team member?

ONE PERSON ON THE SURFACE IN CHARGE

This is very important. There needs to be one person on the surface in the boat who is designated to be in charge of the swim. Conflicts can arise on swims when it is not clear who is in charge. This problem usually occurs at a time when a swimmer is in jeopardy and when a critical decision needs to be made. It's equally important to note that the person in charge can shift and become some other crew member in an emergency. If a swimmer is injured, for example, the on-scene medical expert will take charge. This must be understood and agreed upon by everyone participating. You should address these questions before you begin:

~ Is there training overlap so that if a team member goes down, the swim can still occur?
~ What equipment will each person carry?
~ How will the team communicate?
~ What training should the team conduct together after individual training is complete?
~ How do you handle personality conflicts?

There should be a full dress rehearsal of the swim in conditions as close as possible to those expected on the swim. Even if it is a short thirty-minute swim, it will give the team an opportunity to shake out any last-minute concerns.

SEALs believe the full dress rehearsal should include a casualty drill in which the swimmer is hauled from the water and transported to the door of the nearest appropriate treatment facility. It is important to do the casualty drill so that everyone, including the swimmer, knows what to do. (As a swimmer, I would want to conduct this rehearsal at least two days in advance of my swim, because I don't like to practice getting out of the water. I don't like to practice giving up. I don't like to practice failure. It messes with my head. I want to practice success, but the SEAL says realism is the key.) If done correctly, the casualty drill is as valuable as the swim itself. If multiple methods of pulling the swimmer from the water are available, they should all be tested—boat, Jet Ski, kayak, surfboard. Also rehearse as if other members of the team have gone down. Remember to debrief after the rehearsal.

PLAN FOR THE SWIM/MISSION

Logistics

~ Make a progressive training plan, planned backward from the date/time of the swim.
~ Create a detailed timeline of events—hourly/half hourly—from start to finish.
~ Determine the locations of team members throughout the swim.
~ Plan swim routes.
~ Coordinate transportation—planes, trains, automobiles, boats, Jet Skis, kayaks, etc.
~ Coordinate logistics—how the team will move the equipment.
~ Determine your real financial costs, including possible emergencies.

Food and Fuel

~ Who is in charge of the crew's food, and what is required? Who is in charge of the swimmer's food? Are there specific requirements, such as warming liquids for the swimmer? Who will be feeding the swimmer? How frequently will the swimmer be feeding and how much?

~ How much gasoline is required, and what is the backup for a longer swim or for an emergency?

Medical Considerations

There are swimmers who have died during races and swims from pre-existing medical conditions. L. Tadeus recommends a medical screening—is the swimmer medically capable of swimming? Has the swimmer had a recent physical? A friend of mine had a physical check before his English Channel attempt, and his doctors discovered that his blood pressure was dangerously high from a metabolic condition. Swimming in cold water could have been life threatening. The swimmer had to readjust his goals, swim in warm water, and drop weight, and he has been very successful doing that. Is the crew aware of any possible problems or physical limitations? On one Catalina Channel swim, a swimmer mentioned to her crew that she could see only out of her right eye. In rough conditions, she couldn't change the side of the boat she swam on, to let the boat absorb the rough seas. It also made navigation more difficult for her, and she mentioned that in rough seas, she got seasick. This may have been in part from not being able to see with both eyes, which perhaps affected her balance.

Objectives

The success of a swim may be determined largely by the crew. When selecting a crew, consider what the objectives are of the support team. A good vacation? Money? That warm, fuzzy feeling they get from watching athletes? Camaraderie? Are they focused on the swimmer and the swim or on having a party on the boat? Brief the team thoroughly. Everyone should participate in the brief. Docs should talk medical stuff, boat coxswains should discuss how not to run over a swimmer, and the swimmer should discuss the swim route. Make sure everyone is engaged.

BRIEFING: EXPLAINING THE PLAN

The SEALs have adopted an effective method for briefing missions, and these methods translate well to open water swimming. Note that timing of the briefing is important.

Get the crew together the day or night before the swim and brief them so that you can be sure the entire plan is clear to the support crew and swimmers. This will give the crew and swimmers a chance to discuss and think about the swim and to go over any questions. The brief contains a list of talking points that prompt the person in charge to explain to the crew and swimmer, as well as prompting a discussion that allows everyone to know what he or she is doing to support the swim and the emergency action plan. The brief clarifies details such as in what direction the swimmer will go, the jobs of the crew members, and how often they will serve in a position before being spelled by another crew member.

Things can change before a swim, so it is helpful to have a second briefing an hour or two before the actual swim.

It helps to take a look at the method the SEALs use to plan their missions. Whether they are planning for a training swim or a technically difficult mission with many contingencies, they have developed a clear way to accomplish their objectives, and their experience and techniques can be useful whether you are planning a triathlon, a short ocean swim, or a major channel crossing. I wish I had known about this method when I first began. It would have helped me tremendously in planning and coordinating my swims.

SEAL MISSION PLANNING

The SEALs use three basic ways to conduct mission planning:

1. Well in advance. There is a mission on the horizon that is not at all time-sensitive for which there is plenty of time to plan/train, say, four to six months.

2. Short notice. There is a mission on the immediate horizon that we have trained for but have a short time to bring skills into razor-sharp condition. Think four days from being informed to being on the way to the target.

3. Emergent (implies emergency, as in "it just emerged"). We have four minutes to be out the door and on the way to the target.

L. Tadeus said, "I see a swim 'operation' as something that, if not done regularly in a known location, resides somewhere between situations one and two, above."

PowerPoint is a great planning and briefing tool. Each number below would have its own slide or a group of slides from which to brief and plan. Attached is a sample brief. Notice that it contains a list of talking points that prompt the instructor to engage the trainees in a deeper discussion of the evolution.

Example: Slides that SEAL instructors use to brief a 5.5-nautical-mile swim:

5.5 nm (10.1 km) Swim

Introduction

- Objective: Swim 5.5 nm (10.1 km)
- Emphasis: Proper stroke (underwater recovery) / Buddy cohesiveness / Safety
- Standard: Completion
- NO HANDS OUT OF THE WATER

Equipment

- Personal: Mask/fins/booties/rubber/UDT life jacket w/ flare (day)
- Medical: Ambu
- Comms: See list in comms locker
- Admin: Swim pair lists (2 and 1)
- Marops: Bouys × 2
- Extra gear: Extra mask/fins/booties/UDT life jacket + 1 flare

Execution

- Complete brief
- Inspection
- Muster on beach / Zodiac insert
- WT hit surf
- Swim to buoy / line up
- WT sound off
- Standby for "START"
- Start swim

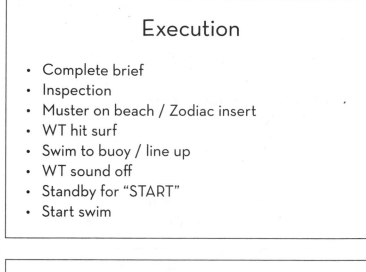

Execution

- At turnaround
  - Sound off with swim pair number, wait to be told to go
  - Swim AROUND buoy
  - Move out
- At end
  - "Swim Pair One, Cake Eater and Smuckatelli"
  - Bottom sample
- Move out (quietly)
- Swim to beach

Contingencies

- Recall: Light on ambu flashing
- Lost Buddy
- Buddy Rescue
- Pickup
  - admin = one hand
  - emergency = one hand waving
  - then whistle, buddy's flare, your flare

Safety Points

- 6-ft (1.8-m) max from buddy
- Watch out for boats
- No air in life jacket

Questions?

STRATEGY

Many channel swimmers and long-distance open water swimmers coordinate their own swims, pay for them, and make the decisions on where they attempt their swims. If they have to wait for favorable conditions but neither the weather nor the tides are cooperating—and they are running out of time, patience, and money—a sense of urgency builds, with an increasing desire to do the swim in poor conditions. The pilot can add to this feeling by encouraging a swimmer to go in less than ideal conditions, since he wants to get paid. Recently, a young swimmer went to England to swim the English Channel. She was waiting through one set of tides and had two swimmers scheduled to go before her. The weather forecast continued to be poor. Her pilot suggested that she swim on a spring tide. To even consider that, she had to be very fast to swim the majority of the twenty-one miles in under six hours and make it to shore before the full force of the tidal change. She also needed to have great weather. Given the weather over the first four days of the neap tide (i.e., tide of minimum range on first and third quarters of the moon), the best times to swim, it did seem likely that the weather would be favorable for the spring tide. She knew that if she could not swim on the neap tide, her option was to swim on the spring, the least favorable time to swim, and risk not succeeding or to wait until the following year for another attempt. She was fortunate that the other swimmers got off, and she was able to attempt her swim, and she completed it in bad conditions. It would have been much better for her—and for other swimmers planning to do a big swim—to designate a "person in charge" of the swim, as the SEALs do.

In the case of open water swimming, the person in charge should be someone who knows the swimmer and her abilities, is involved in the swim, and has some nautical experience. The person in charge needs to be objective in deciding for the swimmer whether a swim is a go or a no-go. The swimmer is the last person who can be objective, due to the cost of the swim and his ego, psychology, and need to see the goal realized.

L. Tadeus said that SEALs recognize that every time you get in the water, you take your life into your own hands. They know that it is far smarter to put your life in someone else's hands—a very competent someone with the resources to pluck you from the jaws of death. We have to take responsibility for the decisions we make; more important, we have to take responsibility for the decisions we don't make. Free will is a bitch. There is always a smarter way to do things, but people are free to do whatever they want. They can be obsessed if they want. They can take meds and swim if they want. They can swim without support if they want. They can ignore all the good advice in the world if they want. They have no one to blame but themselves if they do. The person in charge has to understand the bigger picture. The swimmer focuses on swimming; the person in charge makes decisions and keeps the swimmer safe based on prevailing environmental conditions, and cannot be afraid to say no, even to the swimmer.

Note: The goal of planning is to keep bad things from happening, but you should always plan as though bad things will happen anyway.

BACKUP PLANS

~ What if the water is too cold?
~ What if the water is too warm?
~ What if there is too much boat traffic?
~ What if the waves are too big for the swimmer or the boat?
~ What if the current is too strong?

~ Is there a bump day (a backup day)?

~ Is there a bump location (a backup location)?

SAFETY/OPERATIONAL RISK MANAGEMENT: HOW TO PREVENT MISHAPS AND A FALSE SENSE OF URGENCY

You could encounter multiple risks during a swim. What can you do in advance to mitigate or remove these risks?

Example for open water swimming: risk = hypothermia; mitigation methods = acclimate to colder waters than you'll be swimming in, have rewarming equipment on hand, on-scene medical personnel, and support-team response training.

You can reduce both the probability and the severity of a mishap, depending on which controls (solutions) you implement for each risk. The following diagram is a risk assessment worksheet used by SEAL instructors to assess risks during a 3.5-mile (5.6-kilometer) and a 5.5-mile (8.8-kilometer) open water swim and the controls that they implement to reduce risks.

Risk decisions have to be made at the appropriate level. A SEAL in charge of the second phase of training can authorize training of low and medium risk. His commanding officer can authorize high-risk training and will, if he is confident that the SEAL in charge of second-phase training is taking the necessary precautions. The SEAL in charge of second phase training has to build trust with his commanding officer in order to earn his leadership role in extremely high-risk training.

The SEAL captain in charge of training explained:

A false sense of urgency is the leading cause of mishaps. SEALs who have worked for more than twenty-five years, with the clear view of hindsight, realize

Risk Assessment Worksheet

Training Evolution: 3.5-Mile and 5.5-Mile Swims (Open Water)

Organization:		Date:	Prepared by:				Page 1

Hazards	Probability of Mishap	Effect of Mishap	Risk Level	Controls Implemented	Residual Probability	Residual Effect	Residual Risk Level
Drowning	Seldom (D)	Catastrophic (I)	HIGH	Buddy rule Top-side safety observers Thorough student and instructor safety briefs (EPs and SPs) Student-to-staff communication Emergency Action Plan HM on scene Instructor CPR quals	Unlikely (E)	Catastrophic (I)	MED
Hypoxia	Seldom (D)	Critical (II)	MED	Buddy rule Safety brief Student brief Top-side safety observers Emergency Action Plan HM on scene Trainee fitness	Seldom (D)	Marginal (III)	LOW
Traumatic Injuries	Seldom (D)	Marginal (III)	LOW	Safety brief Student brief Corpsman on scene EVOC on scene Emergency Action Plan	Unlikely (E)	Marginal (III)	LOW

Risk Assessment Worksheet

Training Evolution: 3.5-Mile and 5.5-Mile Swims (Open Water)

Organization:		Date:		Prepared by:		
Shallow Water Blackout	Seldom (D)	Critical (II)	MED	Buddy rule Student-to-instructor communication Instructor-to-student ratio Student brief Safety brief Corpsman on scene Emergency Action Plan Instructor CPR quals Trainees wear inherently buoyant wet suits	Seldom (D)	Marginal (III)	LOW
Boat Traffic	Seldom (D)	Catastrophic (I)	HIGH	Adhere to boat-to-student safety ratio per 2nd phase admin guides Brief boat coxswains on safety precautions Student brief Instructor brief Civilian boat traffic blocked from swimmers Emergency Action Plan thoroughly briefed HM on scene	Unlikely (E)	Catastrophic (I)	MED
Fatigue	Unlikely (E)	Marginal (III)	LOW	Trainee fitness Hydration and nutrition Working schedule shifted to account for high-intensity PT	Unlikely (E)	Negligible (IV)	LOW

Risk Assessment Worksheet
Training Evolution: 3.5-Mile and 5.5-Mile Swims (Open Water)

Organization:			Date:		Prepared by:		
Swimmer-Induced Pulmonary Edema (SIPE)	Seldom (D)	Critical (II)	MED	Trainee fitness Working schedule adjusted to account for high-intensity PT Medical monitoring	Unlikely (E)	Critical (II)	LOW
Lost Swimmer	Seldom (D)	Catastrophic (I)	HIGH	Proper safety-boat-to-student ratio Buddy rule in place Trail and lead instructor with student groups Instructor-to-student ratio shifted in low visibility Safety brief (thorough lost-swimmer procedures) Search procedures GPS onboard to mark last known position Current study	Unlikely (E)	Catastrophic (I)	MED
Dangerous Marine Life	Unlikely (E)	Marginal (III)	LOW	Safety brief Dangerous marine-life class HM on scene	Unlikely (E)	Negligible (IV)	LOW

Risk Assessment Worksheet
Training Evolution: 3.5-Mile and 5.5-Mile Swims (Open Water)

Organization:			Date:	Prepared by:			Page 4
Hypothermia	Seldom (D)	Critical (II)	MED	Check water temps Wet suits when appropriate Medical monitoring—identify students at risk for temperature-related injury HM on scene Swimmer rewarming procedures Swimmer immersion criteria reviewed and on hand	Unlikely (E)	Critical (II)	LOW
Water Quality	Unlikely (E)	Marginal (III)	LOW	Beach and Bay Status Report from NSWC Medical Department Student hygiene briefed by phase HM No swim if water too contaminated or visibility too low	Unlikely (E)	Negligible (IV)	LOW
METOC Conditions	Seldom (D)	Catastrophic (I)	HIGH	No swim if evolution OIC cannot maintain visibility/control of swimmers Increased safety ratio in poor visibility conditions High current taken into consideration for swim course	Unlikely (E)	Catastrophic (I)	MED
High Surf	Seldom (D)	Catastrophic (I)	HIGH	Trainee fitness Swimmer surf-passage training No swim if water safety craft (kayaks/WRVs) cannot traverse surf transit via SD Bay Trainees wear both inherently buoyant wet suits and self-activated life jackets	Unlikely (E)	Catastrophic (I)	MED

Risk Assessment Worksheet
Training Evolution: 3.5-Mile and 5.5-Mile Swims (Open Water)

Organization:		Date:	Prepared by:		
ERV/Ambulance Stuck in Sand	Seldom (D)	Catastrophic (I)	HIGH	Vehicle tires deflated upon entering beach to improve traction Additional vehicle standing by to render assistance Vehicle recovery equipment staged in vehicle Additional vehicle will replace if ERV cannot be recovered to respond to possible emergencies Multiple vehicles used in poor environmental conditions or on long-distance swims	Unlikely (E)	Critical (II)	LOW
Broken/Lost Mask or Fins	Seldom (D)	Marginal (III)	LOW	Extra equipment staged on chase boat for easy access mid-swim Swimmer gear inspection prior to water entry Surf-passage training, practice, brief	Unlikely (E)	Negligible (IV)	LOW

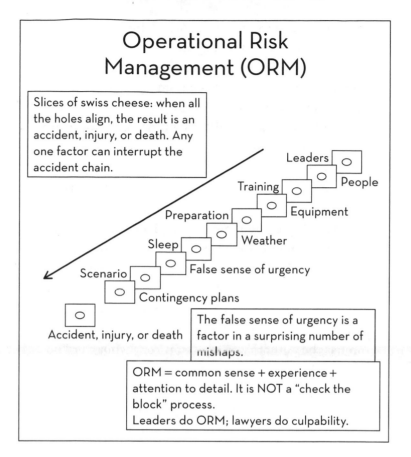

Operational Risk Management (ORM)

Slices of swiss cheese: when all the holes align, the result is an accident, injury, or death. Any one factor can interrupt the accident chain.

Leaders

People

Training

Equipment

Preparation

Weather

Sleep

False sense of urgency

Scenario

Contingency plans

Accident, injury, or death

The false sense of urgency is a factor in a surprising number of mishaps.

ORM = common sense + experience + attention to detail. It is NOT a "check the block" process.
Leaders do ORM; lawyers do culpability.

that many of the accidents, injuries, or deaths that occurred during their time with the teams were preventable.

The diagram above depicts a series of swiss cheese slices, with each slice corresponding to a distinct factor, including training, preparation, people, leadership, weather, et cetera. When a hole in each slice lines up with the next, that's an accident chain starting. When the holes line up from start to finish, that's an accident chain occurring. Any one slice can be pulled out and the chain is broken, preventing the occurrence of the accident. The interesting thing is that one single factor is present in an overwhelming number of accidents: a false sense of urgency. This false sense of urgency— miscalculation of actual time versus perceived time available—is present in so many accidents that it has to be something worth studying.

With the SEALs, risk management plans are the leader's business (this information applies to the person in charge of an open water swim). It is *not* a "check the block" paperwork drill. Good risk assessment and management is equal parts leadership, experience, and attention to detail.

As an added risk management requirement, the SEALs appoint one person to an event who can interrupt a fatality by stepping back and looking at the scenario with an unbiased eye. That's why they have one leader in each phase of training or a race who stands back from the event. That person has the requisite clarity of view to see the details, understand the big picture, and step in to prevent an accident. That person has the authority to say "stop" or "whoa" or "no" and, in doing so, prevent an accident. This method directly applies to open water swimming. It would certainly make sense to have this person connected with an open swimming race or on board during an open water swim.

As a SEAL captain shares, "Life is not a risk-free event. Risk is actually fun and what drives many people to enjoy life. But calculated risk is the opposite of gambling. The SEALs are trained to calculate risk and make sound decisions. Navy Special Warfare doesn't train gamblers. SEALs are trained to calculate risk and make sound judgments."

EMERGENCY ACTION PLAN: WHO IS NOTIFIED IN ADVANCE AND HOW TO REACH THEM DURING THE SWIM

Use an emergency action plan: what to do in the event of a mishap. Ask the following questions:

~ What are all the possible injuries? This includes both the support team and the swimmer. If something can happen, however remote the chance, plan for it. Murphy is out there, enforcing his law.

~ What is the immediate treatment for each?

~ Is immediate-treatment equipment with the support team?

~ What is the extended treatment for each?

~ Is anyone on scene qualified to provide immediate aid for any injury?

~ Where are the nearest treatment facilities for major injuries?

~ How do you get to treatment facilities from the location you are swimming in?

~ What is the nearest identifiable location, if you are relying on 911, that an ambulance can use to meet or locate you?

~ Have you staged an ambulance onshore?

~ Do you know the numbers for LifeFlight and a good location for them to land?

~ How do you communicate with them? By megaphone? Hand signals?

~ Do treatment facilities accept the swimmer/team members' insurance?

~ If you are relying on the USCG, what are their go/no-go criteria for coming to save the swimmer? They'll do the best they can, but if someone goes swimming during a hurricane, he may end up taking responsibility for his actions at the expense of his own life.

COMPLETION OF SWIM AND REWARMING

~ Plan the best you can.

~ Conduct the swim with what you have.

~ Execute the rewarming plan (if required).

~ Execute medical testing (if required).

DEBRIEFING

If a swim requires this level of planning, then it requires debriefing. Rehearsals require debriefing, too. Everyone should sit down and discuss what went right and what went wrong. If something went went wrong, discussion should ensue about what caused it. Recommendations should follow on how to keep it from going wrong in the future. *Document, document, document.* If you don't record it, it didn't happen. Given enough time, all the experience and lessons learned will fade away unless there is a way to review them. For a swim you are doing the first time but intend to repeat using what you have learned, you can go from months of planning down to minutes with the right team and the right swimmer on future swims.

FURTHER SEAL ADVICE WHEN PLANNING A SWIM

You may have specific questions for organizing an open water swim. For instance, how do you determine if a pilot is qualified? How do you know if the boat you are using has been inspected and will operate safely? What kind of aid equipment do you need on the support boat? How would you rehearse before a swim? How would you check the weather forecast before a swim? Do you write down the crew's roles and responsibilities so they know precisely what they will be doing during a swim?

There are specific training certificates for seamanship and boat handling. For example, L. Tadeus has certificates for training in F-470 Zodiac, 25-foot (7.6-meter) Boston Whaler, 11-meter rigid inflatable boat, 25-foot aluminum-hull skiff, outboard motor repair, CPR (Red Cross), basic lifesaving, marine radio operator's permit, and inland and international rules of the road. He is also licensed in numerous types of sailing, inboard and outboard vessels up to two hundred tons near coastal by International Yacht Training through the Maritime Institute in Point Loma, California. The licenses are recognized in twenty-two different countries. He recommends looking for coast guard (USCG) licenses as well. Anyone can buy a boat; no certificates or licenses are required unless the boat is made available for charter. It is not enough to be qualified.

A pilot should also be current. L. Tadeus keeps a sea log every time he goes out on a boat, the same way he keeps a dive log every time he goes underwater, a demo log every time he blows something up, and an air log every time he jumps out of a plane. The point is, a qualified pilot should have documentation of his experience, both volume and currency. Any pilot who doesn't have such documentation probably isn't worth the effort.

To check out the boat, do a self-inspection and ask for records of inspections by reputable authorities. If a boat has not been inspected by the U.S. Coast Guard, you probably won't want to hire it for support for an open water swim. Here is a list of the aid equipment you need to check for on a boat: floatation devices, their locations markers (GPS, EPIRB), and boat hooks. Is there anything on board that would help a struggling swimmer until physical aid could be rendered? Look to see if the boat has a swimmer cutout or a ladder. Does the boat have a positively buoyant spine board to cross-deck a swimmer from boat to boat or boat to pier? Is the setup of the boat suitable for a swim? If the boat was originally set up for fishing, does it have a diving platform to assist the crew and swimmer when needed during the swim? It is also important to determine fuel costs before your swim. It can cost up to fifteen hundred dollars to fill up a decent-sized vessel—a forty-foot Sport Fisher, for example—no small cost. The overriding concern is whether the boat can carry enough fuel to run engines and generators at slow speeds for many hours and still have enough to handle contingencies and mishaps.

NOAA is the ultimate authority on weather, but their forecasts can be very general. There are local weather sources that are much more specific for a given area. USCG publishes local weather advisories on specific MARBAND channels every few minutes for moment-to-moment changes. Note that USCG publishes a Notice to Mariners (NOTAMS) that gives updates to local hydrographic changes; this is a good source to consult for official local knowledge on physical oceanographic conditions.

There is a lot of value in writing down roles and responsibilities for the pilot and each crew member. Your crew may need some advice on how to organize, direct, supervise, and lead a support team. While some roles and responsibilities may overlap slightly, roles should be well understood and distinct for efficiency's sake during mishap response—being able to respond when something goes wrong.

The SEALs rehearse everything they can before a mission. It is equally wise to do this before a swim. There were times when I did not like the situation surrounding a rehearsal. Before my swim in Antarctica, the ship's doctor suddenly decided that the crew and I needed to rehearse my being pulled out of the water. He wanted me to act like I had experienced cardiac arrest, and have my crew put me on a stretcher and carry me up the ship's stairs. What the doctor was asking me to do was to rehearse my death. If you jump into extremely cold water, there is a chance that you can overstimulate your vagus nerve and cause your heart to stop.

For two years I had trained specifically for the swim in Antarctica, and I had psychologically prepared for it. I believed it would be possible to swim a mile in 32-degree F (0-degree C) water in a swimsuit, swim cap, and goggles. I had planned out the swim in my mind and how it would unfold—I didn't want to rehearse my death. It was the opposite of everything I had been doing to prepare myself. I told the doctor that I could not participate in the drill, that another member of my crew had offered to take my place. None of it made sense, because the ship's crew had already developed a quick and efficient way of extracting people from the water and getting them onto the ship. They pulled the victim into the Zodiac and, with a crane, lifted the Zodiac with the victim onto the ship's bow and then carried the victim to a room where the ship's doctor could attend to the victim.

The ship's doctor wanted to try something new. My crew rehearsed with him. One crew member was placed on a stretcher and tied down. Three to four members of the crew tried to lift the stretcher and carry her up the ship's stairs, but the angle was too steep and they nearly dropped the stretcher, with her on it, into the water three times. I was glad I didn't participate in the drill, which occurred only an hour before my swim. Now, as I look back on it with the SEALs' input, I see that there's a lot of value to be gained from using the actual swimmer in a mishap drill. If I had to do it again, I would participate in the casuality drill—but a few days, not hours, before my swim.

MEDICAL CHECK BEFORE SWIM

It is very important to have a swimmer medically checked out before a swim. There are medical conditions that preclude extreme swimming (hole in the heart), medical conditions that require adjustment of swim conditions (blood pressure), and conditions that could increase risk without mitigation (one blind eye).

When I was planning my open water swims, often my crew and I would discuss the plan for a year. When we reached the location for the start of the swim, where I would train for a week or two, we would discuss, question, and go over details. We would spend hours thinking and refining ideas. And just before the swim, we would go over the plan—the brief—again. Because we'd discussed our plan so many times, it did not take long to brief the crew. I asked L. Tadeus how he determines the amount of time to be devoted to a brief.

The complexity of the swim drives the complexity of the brief. For SEALs doing a pool dive, the brief is a five-minute conversation. A sixty-two-man trainee dive using contract dive vessels takes three excruciatingly thorough briefs to trainees, instructors, and boat crews, covering a total of about three hours using PowerPoint.

It's unlikely that a swimmer will have access to his own emergency response vehicle. But if a swimmer has access to support vessels, he may also have access to an emergency response vehicle. In either case, the boat has to get the swimmer to a location where he can link up with an emergency response vehicle for follow-on transport to a medical facility.

Providing that both the boat and the ambulance can get to a common location, how do you direct the ambulance to that spot? Most piers don't have an address. If the location is remote, then you are looking at Air Evac. Do you know anyone who is capable of assessing a helicopter landing zone and talking the bird to that location? We can do this in five minutes, but we rehearse it. In a situation where seconds are crucial, there's not much time to figure it out on the fly.

The bottom line is: The swim route isn't the only route you need to think out in advance. Despite an inspection, a boat can break down. SEALs do at least a cursory inspection to tell whether a boat is obviously near breakdown or in good shape, but the rest is in fate's hands. Boats break. That's what they seem designed to do. There should be a contingency plan in place: Two is one, one is none.

RECOMMENDATIONS FOR LONG TRAINING SWIMS AND DOCUMENTATION

Recently, Erez Israeli contacted me from Israel. He was starting to train for a ten-mile swim in the Sea of Galilee. He'd learned to swim only two years before. He had run a couple of marathons and competed in some full-length triathlons. He said, "I need to try something interesting. Something that will be challenging and keep me in shape." He asked me to help him with his training and preparation for a long-distance swim. He needed assistance with his stroke, and he listened to my suggestion to film a video of his swimming. He sent it to a stroke technician who analyzed his stroke and gave him pointers. Erez worked with Dani Jaituv, a top swimmer and coach in Israel. Dani helped with his speed and endurance. Erez coordinated boat support with swimming friends in Israel.

Erez called me the week before, a couple of days before, and the evening before his swim to ask for any additional advice. I suggested that he pack his swim bag at least a couple of days before his swim and go through a checklist of the things he would need: at least one extra swimsuit, pair of goggles, and swim cap; two or three towels for himself; skin lubricant; and anything he thought he needed for the swim, including food, water bottles, and other fluids he planned to drink during his swim. Even though he would be swimming in the Sea of Galilee and the water and air would be warm, I suggested that he bring warm clothes, because once he stopped exercising, he would stop producing heat, and the cooled blood beneath his skin would circulate to his core and drop his temperature. I suggested that he have water shoes, flip-flops, or aqua socks that he could put on at the end of the swim, in case there were freshwater clamshells or broken glass on the sand when he was climbing to shore. I also suggested that he wear clear goggles in the dark and smoked or tinted goggles during the day to protect his eyes from UVA and UVB rays. I sent him the following advice specific to the swim:

1. Feed Every Twenty Minutes to Every Half Hour

    ~ Try warm fluids. [If he'd been training for a hot-water swim, I would have suggested cold fluids.]
    ~ See which fluids work best for you during a swim. Limit this test to two kinds of fluids during each training swim.
    ~ See which foods work best for you during a swim. Limit the test to one or two types of solid foods.
    ~ Have your crew record what you are eating, how much, and how frequently.
    ~ Make your feedings brief so you stay warm.
    ~ Try to feed quickly to maintain your body heat.

2. Have Your Support Crew Take Your Stroke Rate Every Half Hour, Before They Stop You to Feed
    This way they can get you at your pace, not when you're slowing to feed.

3. Have Your Pilot Plot Your Progress on the Navigational Chart and Indicate the Distance You Have Swum and Your Speed Every Half Hour

4. Have the Pilot Indicate Wind Speed and Direction Every Half Hour and Note It on a Chart or in a Log

5. Have the Pilot Indicate Current Speed and Direction and Note Them in a Log
    The SEAL observed, "They better be doing this anyway—it's important from an evidentiary perspective in case they run aground or sink."

6. Have Your Crew Evaluate You During Your Feedings

They need to make sure you aren't going into hypothermia (or hyperthermia, during a hot-water swim). They need to look at your shoulders and lips and make sure they aren't bluish in color. They need to look at your fingers at the beginning of the swim and see the way you normally swim and then check to see if they are spreading apart. If you can't keep your fingers together as you normally do, your brain may be cooling down and you might be losing fine motor control. L. Tadeus suggested, "Have your crew ask you questions that will make you think, such as, 'What was the day three days ago?'" He also recommended: "Have your crew ask you, 'How are you feeling?' You need to be able to respond, 'I feel fine.' If you can't say that phrase or can't articulate it clearly, then you may be going into hypothermia." If you are swimming in a desert environment and the air temperature is hot and the water is seventy-five degrees, make sure you're drinking enough fluids and you aren't overheating. Your crew should be aware if you are excreting fluid; if you aren't, you probably aren't drinking enough fluid.

During the brief feeding stops, your support crew will ask how you are feeling. It is important to record it, because when the swim is completed, you can pinpoint when you were feeling good and when things were tough. After the swim is completed, you can look at these points and figure out if there is a way to improve. Here are some of the questions you can ask yourself: Do I need to do more workout swims in rougher conditions? Was I tired because I need to train more intensely, or was my blood sugar low and I needed more food or fluid? Did I lose my mental focus? Did I doubt my ability to complete the swim?

Look at your workouts that led up to the swim and see where you can improve. You might need to add more intensity to your workouts or stroke work, or focus more on pace. By going the distance in water conditions similar to those of your big swim, you will strengthen yourself mentally and physically, and you will be more prepared for your next swim.

7. Apply at Least Three Layers of Sunscreen Before You Swim

In open water, you need to prevent sunburn. Apply the first layer of waterproof sunscreen at least two hours before your swim, then apply a second coating an hour and a half before, and a third layer at least an hour before you swim. You may want to have a friend apply the sunscreen, especially on your back. If you apply it yourself, wear surgical gloves or wash your hands well with soap and water so you don't get any sunscreen on your goggles.

8. Visually Record Your Swim

Keep a written and video record of your swim.

Erez completed his first ten-mile swim in the Sea of Galilee. His crew recorded the swim, and he was able to go over the information with his support crew and coach, figuring out what worked and what didn't. He made corrections, adjusted his workouts and his stroke, worked on his speed and pace, and a few months later, with a strong and knowledgeable support crew, he swam the length of the Sea of Galilee, a thirteen-mile swim in a straight line, though he swam closer to fifteen miles.

After that success, he planned to swim across the Catalina Channel, but during his health check, his physician told him that it was not healthy for him to carry the extra weight he'd need to insulate him from the cold on the Catalina swim or in the English Channel. He was tremendously disappointed. He said he gave himself an hour to be upset and then put it in perspective. He realized that the reason he was swimming was to be healthy, and he would not be healthy if he carried extra weight. He took my suggestion and changed his goal to long-distance warm-water swims.

He found a group of qualified support people and friends who helped him and guided him. He swam the length of the Sea of Galilee twice—a distance of 26.2 miles (42.1 kilometers)—in 75-degree F (23.8-degree C) water, in a time of eighteen hours and fifty-one minutes. He accomplished a long-distance swim off Croatia, has set new open water goals, and is now training for a double-length triathlon.

Chapter 13

Dangerous Marine Organisms

This chapter applies to all levels of open water swimmers. There are many dangerous marine animals in the world's oceans, and there are volumes written by physicians and biologists. The goal for this section is to highlight some of the most dangerous and most encountered animals and to include up-to-date treatments advised by physicians who are experts in this area.

Warnings that your parents gave you as a child, "Watch where you step" and "Look but don't touch," should be heeded in the ocean environment, especially in tropical waters. Some of the most beautiful sea animals produce powerful and even life-threatening stings or bites. These animals may also pose a problem on the beach.

A few years ago, when a friend invited me to swim off the remote islands of Fiji, I researched the area and talked to local Fijians before I went swimming. They pointed out the animals I should avoid, and I went for a long warm swim on the shore side of a coral reef. The water was transparent turquoise, delightfully warm, and teeming with life. There were so many beautiful alien-shaped sea animals and brilliant-colored fish. It was one of the most fun and fascinating swims that I ever had.

When I climbed out of the water, the palm trees were swaying slowly in the heavy, humid breeze. I went for a long beach walk and met a couple of local Fijians from the small village nearby. They noticed that I was barefoot and asked why I wasn't wearing water shoes on the beach. They said that with the tidal change, small poisonous sea snakes often get left in tiny pools of water on the beach, and they bite. Visitors should wear water shoes.

RESEARCH SEMITROPICAL AND TROPICAL WATERS BEFORE SWIMMING

Before entering freshwater lakes, ponds, streams, and rivers, talk with locals about animals and fish that might cause health concerns or problems.

This was something that Beverly Johnson taught me. Beverly was known for her expertise as a world-class rock climber and mountaineer; she also worked on documentary films all around the world. She traveled to Queensland, Australia, to work on a project connected with the Great Barrier Reef. She was staying at a hotel in Darwin near a river. It was summer and extremely hot and humid, and she longed to go for a swim. She asked the hotel manager if she could swim in the river, and he said she could, but the way he answered made her feel uneasy, and she thought he might be teasing her. She asked for more information. The manager explained that there were no restrictions on swimming in the river, but he wouldn't do it. He said there were crocodiles that lounged on the riverbanks and fed in the river. Beverly decided to forgo the river swim.

The following marine animals are dangerous, and swimmers should do their best to avoid them.

BRISTLE WORMS

Bristle worms are annelid worms. Each segment of the bristle worm has a pair of fleshy protrusions called parapodia, and these contain numerous bristles called chaetae, which are made of chitin. There are more than ten thousand species of bristle worms found in all waters frequented by swimmers and divers. There are bristle worms that live in the coldest ocean temperatures of the abyssal plain, tolerate the extreme high temperatures near hydrothermal vents, are found at all depths of the ocean, and are also found in fresh water.

Bristle worms are often brightly colored and multicolored; they may be iridescent or even luminescent. Most bristle worms are under four inches in length, though some may reach up to almost ten feet. When a worm is stimulated, its body contracts and the bristles are erected. The bristles can penetrate skin like cactus thorns and are very difficult to remove. Some marine worms are also able to inflict painful bites and may cause a burning sensation or a red itchy rash. These occur most often on the hands and fingers. Untreated, the pain usually disappears after a few hours, but the itching and swelling may last two to three days.

Paul Auerbach, MD, MS, is the Redlich Family Professor of Surgery in the Division of Emergency Medicine at Stanford University School of Medicine and an expert in wilderness medicine and on marine animal stings. He wrote the book *Medicine for the Outdoors, 5th Edition* (see Sources for website address; page 301). In his book, Dr. Auerbach covers a much wider range of marine animals and other medical treatments. For this manual I focused on the marine animals that swimmers are likely to encounter.

Treatment for Bristle Worms

Dr. Auerbach gave the following recommendations for treating bristle worm stings: Remove all large visible bristles with tweezers. Then gently dry the skin, taking care to avoid breaking or further embedding the spines. Apply a layer of adhesive tape, rubber cement, or a facial peel to remove the residual smaller spines. If the inflammation is significant, the victim may benefit from the administration of topical hydrocortisone 1 percent lotion.

CORAL REEFS

Part of the reason many of us swim in the open water is to have unique experiences, to see parts of the world that we could never see from land. Some of my most pleasurable swims and dives have been around coral reefs off Australia, Fiji, Egypt, Israel, Jordan, South Africa, Hawaii, and the Out Islands in the Bahamas. There's nothing like swimming through warm transparent waters, seeing a world teeming with colorful clown, angel- and triggerfish hovering above the coral recesses. It is mesmerizing to watch soft corals swaying in the ocean currents, and the blue iridescent-mantled clams slowly opening and 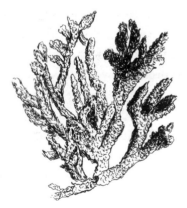 closing their giant shells, and schools of silvery fish swirling by. Swimming above coral reefs is like entering giant aquariums without walls.

One of the world's experts on coral reefs, Cindy Hunter, a biologist at the University of Hawaii, appreciates the vast beauty of the reefs but recognizes an equal significance:

Besides being thrilling to swim over, coral reefs also form the base of the food chain around tropical coastlines. This is where animals, microbes, and plants mingle, creating relationships that scientists are still figuring out. Corals themselves house tiny golden-brown algae inside their own cells, and use the carbohydrates produced by their "housemates" for energy to build their skeletons. These hard skeletons of coral colonies give myriad other reef creatures places to shelter and forage for food. Some parrot fish crunch up coral skeletons with their strong front teeth, pooping out tons of new sand each year. When life gets stressful (as when global warming results in water temperatures higher than about two degrees above the summer norm), the corals eject the algae, resulting in ghostly pale reefs—also known as coral belching—which may take many months to recover, if at all.

The coral reefs off Hawaii are comprised of compact colonies of many identical individual "polyps." The individual polyps secrete calcium carbonate and form a hard skeleton and create colonies that comprise a reef. Some corals use stinging cells on their tentacles to catch plankton. Corals reproduce by spawning, using day length and moon phases to synchronize the release of eggs and sperm. Finger corals reproduce near midnight, just after the full moon, while others, such as rice corals, spawn for a few hours after sunset at the new moon during the summer months.

Cindy teaches a minicourse at the University of Hawaii called Romance on the Reef in which students can watch the corals spawn to create new reefs. She says there are more than sixty species in Hawaii that vary in size, shape, and color. Corals are nature's most exquisite underwater sculptures. The reefs serve as natural barricades to ocean waves and protect the Hawaiian Islands as well as other landmasses from erosion.

Cindy advised me not to get too close to the coral while

swimming. She explained that the coral is sharp and rigid and can scrape and cut the skin, and a coral cut may become easily infected. She also advised me not to walk on the reef. Coral is fragile and can break off easily. It may take a full year for some species of coral to regrow an inch.

Always talk with the lifeguards and local people about the water and reef conditions. Tidal changes have a large impact on the reef and on safety. Calm blue waters can be deceptive.

Mark, a friend who is a beach lifeguard and a top open water swimmer, traveled with his wife to Hawaii for a vacation. The water was sparkling blue and calm, and the tide was high when they swam out to investigate the reef. They'd gotten caught up in the surrounding beauty when Mark suddenly noticed that the tide was moving out. The waves were breaking on the exposed reef and growing larger as the tide moved farther out. Mark realized that they had to swim toward land to avoid being slammed onto the reef by the waves. He watched the swells, found a lull in the waves, and managed to get his wife in safely, but he sustained scrapes and cuts from the coral.

Even small coral and barnacle cuts can become very serious. Tropical waters contain considerable numbers of uncommon (on land) bacteria, and cuts can rapidly become infected, sometimes with these germs.

David Yudovin learned this during a first crossing in Indonesia from Pulau Tanah Masa to Pulau Pini. When he was close to shore, he swam over a coral reef where the water was stagnant and very warm (92 degrees F, or 33.3 degrees C). He nicked his foot on the coral and didn't think anything of it, but the water was full of bacteria, and within hours his foot swelled and a staphylococcus (staph) infection started traveling up his leg. His temperature rose to 104 degrees F. He tried the local antibiotics manufactured in Jakarta, but they were not as potent as the antibiotics manufactured in the United States. Though they held the infection back, he realized he needed to get home to see his doctor and obtain more potent medications. It has taken him three months to heal and feel normal again.

Infections from coral cuts or cuts from shellfish are not unusual in tropical waters. A friend who has been involved in outrigger canoeing for years once told me that many tropical islands do not have sewage treatment facilities and that human waste drains directly into the ocean. Know where the sewage drains are located, and the current water movements around the islands, to avoid swimming in contaminated water.

You may want to consult your primary care or travel medicine practitioner before you leave on your trip, and find out if it's possible to obtain a prescription for antibiotics and instructions to carry with you in case they are needed.

Treatment for Coral and Barnacle Cuts

L. Tadeus describes barnacles as underwater razor blades. If you are cut by coral or barnacles, Dr. Paul Auberbach recommends:

~ Seek medical treatment at once if the cuts are severe or if there are any signs of infection.
~ If you suffer small scrapes or cuts, scrub them with soap and water, then thoroughly wash with fresh disinfected water.
~ If the wound is causing a stinging sensation, rinse it briefly with vinegar. This should help reduce the stinging. Be sure to rinse the vinegar completely from the wound.
~ Flush the cut or scrape with a mixture of one-half water and one-half medicinal over-the-counter hydrogen peroxide to remove coral fragments, then flush the wound with fresh disinfected water.
~ Wash the wound daily. Apply bacitracin or another similar antiseptic ointment three to four times per day.

Coral cuts are notorious for becoming infected. Check the coral cuts at least once a day to see if they are becoming inflamed, swollen, red, or tender. If the wound develops into a festering sore or an ulcer with drainage, or if redness spreads on the skin around the wound area, seek immediate medical attention.

FIRE CORAL

Fire coral is a marine animal that can sting in a manner similar to that of jellyfish. It is widely distributed in tropical and subtropical waters, and swimmers and divers often mistake it for seaweed. Fire corals have tiny stinging cells. Once when I was off the Bahamas learning how to snorkel, my leg brushed up against a patch of fire coral. The sting burned, but it did not cause shortness of breath, swelling tongue, or tightness in my chest, which would have signified an allergic reaction. I followed the advice of medical experts, who recommend the following:

~ Rinse the affected area with salt water, then apply vinegar to the sting area (isopropyl alcohol works equally well).
~ Check the sting area for tiny adherent fragments. If there are any, remove them with tweezers.
~ Check the wound daily. If it is inflamed but not infected (you may need a medical expert to make this determination), apply hydrocortisone cream two or three times a day to reduce itching, and apply alcohol to prevent infection.

Dr. Auerbach also recommends using citrus (for example, fresh lime) juice that contains citric, malic, or tartaric acid.

JELLYFISH

Jellyfish are commonly known as jellies or sea jellies. They inhabit every ocean and live in depths ranging from surface waters to the ocean's greatest depths. Members of the jellyfish family that are of concern to swimmers include fire coral, hydroids, sea wasps, and anemones.

There are more than fifteen hundred species of jellyfish, and they are exquisitely designed animals. Some have clear transparent domes and tentacles, while others are opaque and multicolored. With their tentacles splayed out, jellyfish often resemble flowers. They move slowly, rhythmically, and gracefully as they pulsate through the water. They range in size from barely visible to the human eye to over three feet in diameter. Some jellyfish, such as certain moon jellies, do not sting, while others produce powerful stings that can be potentially dangerous or even life threatening.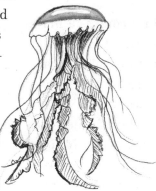

A jellyfish sting occurs when a person comes in contact with the tentacles or appendages. The jellyfish inject toxins into the swimmer's skin. These toxins can cause stings that range in severity from a mild burning sensation and redness to excruciating pain and severe blistering of the skin. Symptoms may include nausea, vomiting, shortness of breath, and muscle spasms. Jellyfish don't have to be intact to produce stings. Tentacles that break off the animal and float in the open water, surf, or on the beach may retain their potency for months.

Before entering any natural body of water, check with the local fishermen, swimmers, lifeguards, surfers, boaters, coast guard, divers, navy, marine biologists, or any other people who might know if there are jellyfish in the area.

There are often times of the year and places in the world where jellyfish are more prevalent. In many areas that have been overfished, there are greater numbers of jellyfish.

Kelly Gleason is a maritime archaeologist and an open water swimmer who swims and dives off Hawaii and monitors the jellyfish populations. She noted two types that are problematic in Hawaii. The first is the man-of-war—but be advised that what people in Hawaii call the man-of-war jellyfish is a different species from the larger jellyfish of the same common name, typically found in the Atlantic in the summertime. The Atlantic Ocean version is quite hazardous.

In Hawaii, the man-of-war are tiny purple creatures approximately the size of golf balls, with long, stringy tentacles. Gleason said, "Most of the time it is the floating tentacles that get people. They can feel razor-sharp, but the sting is usually temporary, and I've always managed them okay. Some people scar really badly from them, but that is just an individual thing. They tend to accumulate on the windward and south sides of Oahu and can be seasonal (worse in the fall, when winds are strong on the windward side), but you can run into them at any time."

The second species of jellyfish that keep people out of the Hawaiian waters are the box jellyfish. Gleason said,

People who are really careful about them will stay out of the water when they are around. They arrive ten days after a full moon, so they can be predicted. Places with heavy tourism, like Hanauma Bay, close when the box jellies are out. The stings are really bad and can send you to the hospital. I've heard stories of people getting stung and then needing assistance to get back in to shore. When box jellies are out, if they are bad, you will see them washed up onshore. That is a way we can tell if it is a few days after the ten-day window. It's best to check the shoreline and always best to be conservative. The lifeguards are pretty well versed in jellyfish and particularly box jellies, so lifeguards are always a good source of info if you should go in the water.

Prevention of Jellyfish Stings

To prevent stings, find out if jellyfish are prevalent in the area that day. If they are, swim in a different area.

There are a number of Australian swimmers and surfers who wear "sting" suits or "stinger" suits. The sting suits are made from Lycra, and the Aussies say that they block most stingers. Sting suits may also help to reduce sun exposure, though they may also increase the chances of chafing. Apply BodyGlide, Vaseline, or another type of lubrication to the inseams and areas of the garment that may cause chafing, especially around the neck.

Some swimmers may opt to wear a nylon-rubber dive skin, but if you are swimming in warm waters, make sure that you do not become overheated, and drink sufficient fluids to avoid dehydration.

There is also a jellyfish sting protective lotion, Safe Sea (see Sources for website address; page 301), with and without sun block, with a barrier cream that blocks or diminishes the stings of many jellyfish species.

Treatment for Jellyfish Stings

The physical reaction to jellyfish stings depends on the species of jellyfish and on a swimmer's sensitivity to the stings. The most immediate danger is an acute, severe allergic reaction: A mild allergic response of itching and skin hives can suddenly transform into anaphylactic shock, which includes a substantial drop in blood pressure, facial and airway swelling, difficulty breathing, collapse, and sometimes death.

Most beach lifeguards and surf lifesavers are aware of the species of jellyfish in their area and know how to treat these stings. However, this is not always the case. On a warm summer day a few years ago, my friend Martha was off the shores of Martha's Vineyard and swam into a jellyfish that wrapped its tentacles around her arms, injecting venom from its stinging cells into her skin and causing extreme pain. Martha managed to climb out of the water and walk to the lifeguard station, where she asked the lifeguards to treat her stings. Unfortunately, they didn't know what to do and did not have any remedies. She took a hot shower, which increased her pain.

There are differing opinions or controversy about the most effective treatments for jellyfish stings. This situation became clear when Sandy from California was swimming a long distance off Hawaii. She was stung by a man-of-war. She said it was very painful, but she was only halfway through her swim and didn't want to stop. Her crew told her that the best treatment for the jellyfish stings was uric acid, which would supposedly break down the jellyfish's stinging cells and reduce her pain. One of the men on board her support boat offered to urinate on her arms. It should be noted that urine is not composed of uric acid; furthermore, it has never been shown to be an effective topical remedy for jellyfish stings. She accepted the treatment, but it was extremely difficult to apply the liquid. She was bobbing up and down in the water, and he was rocking back and forth on the boat, attempting to urinate on her. Somehow he managed to hit the target with undiluted urine. However, the pain didn't diminish, and she decided to continue swimming—until another man-of-war zapped her across the face. Her friend immediately offered his help again, but she wisely declined and climbed out of the water.

Some people claim that jellyfish toxins can build up in the body if a swimmer is stung multiple times. This is unproved. It is possible that a person who is repetitively stung over a period of a few hours might retain toxin that circulates in the bloodstream. An allergic reaction may be immediate or slightly delayed, and there are different allergic reactions that confuse

> Topical lidocaine 4 percent also may effectively numb a jellyfish sting but may not lessen the envenomation.

the picture. A mild allergic reaction can be a warning that the situation might soon deteriorate, so the victim should be watched closely until there is a clear trend toward improvement.

Dr. Paul Auerbach wrote that, depending on the species, size, geographic location, time of year, and other natural factors, the toxins in the jellyfish's stinging cells can cause stings that range in severity from a mild burning sensation and redness around the sting sites to excruciating pain and severe blistering of the skin. The stings can cause nausea, vomiting, shortness of breath, and muscle spasms. Jellyfish toxins affect people differently, and treatment for one jellyfish species may work well for that species but may not be effective for another species. The treatment for the Atlantic man-of-war jellyfish, for example, is different from the treatment for the man-of-war jellyfish off the shores of Hawaii.

BOX JELLYFISH

Box jellyfish belong to the class Cuboazoa. They are cube- or umbrella-shaped, and differ from the true jellyfish, Scyphozoa, which are dome- or crown-shaped. Many box jellyfish are transparent and pale blue, making them difficult to see in the water. They do not simply pulsate and drift through the water column, as do "true" jellyfish, to find food. Box jellyfish are believed to hunt their prey and are among the most venomous animals in the world. Stings from *Chironex fleckeri, Carukia barnesi*, and *Malo kingi* are extremely painful. A sting from *Chironex fleckeri* may cause death in a matter of minutes from shock, cessation of breathing, and abnormal heart rhythms.

Chironex fleckeri, Carukia barnesi, and *Malo kingi* are largely found off northern Australia and the tropical Indo-Pacific Ocean. Other species of box jellyfish are found in tropical and subtropical oceans, including the subtropical and tropical waters of the Atlantic Ocean and east Pacific

Ocean, with some species found as far north as California, the Mediterranean, Japan, South Africa, and New Zealand.

Australians have discovered that the species *Chironex fleckeri* is particularly dangerous during the wet season, from roughly November to April off northern Australia. This box jellyfish is the largest in the species, measuring up to about one foot, or thirty centimeters, in diameter, with tentacles that stretch up to nine feet, or three meters, long. *Carukia barnesi*, the other dangerous species of box jellyfish, is tiny, the size of a thumbnail, and also found in waters off Australia. It is commonly known as Irukandji. Stings from this species cause muscle spasm, nausea and vomiting, sweating, high blood pressure, and sometimes death.

Treatment for Box Jellyfish Stings

Dr. Auerbach recommended the following treatment for a sting from *Chironex fleckeri*, the box jellyfish:

~ Immediately pour vinegar (5 percent acetic acid) over the sting sites.
~ Keep the swimmer as still as possible, and continue saturating the sting area with vinegar, until a physician attends to the person.
~ If you are out at sea or on an isolated shore, let the vinegar remain on the skin and tentacles for ten minutes to attain its full neutralizing effect. Then remove the tentacles with tweezers.

Lifeguards in Australia are qualified to give an intramuscular injection of antivenom to the sting victim onsite if needed.

Treatment for Pacific and Atlantic Man-of-War

Dr. Auerbach recommended the following treatment for stings from any Portuguese man-of-war (Atlantic version or

Pacific version: "bluebottle"), Irukandji, fire coral, stinging hydroid, sea nettle, or sea anemone: Use vinegar or rubbing alcohol to saturate the skin, or apply soaked compresses. Some authorities advise against using alcohol because it has not been proved effective beyond a doubt; however, many people believe it is a good alternative to vinegar. For some jellyfish stings, people have found household ammonia or a slurry of baking soda to be effective. Different species of jellyfish carry different toxins and produce different reactions to their stings. It is extremely important to know ahead of time what will work for the stings in the area where you are swimming.

If a topical decontaminant, such as vinegar, is not available, then rinse the skin with seawater. Do not rinse the skin with fresh water, and do not apply ice directly to the skin. This may cause more stinging cells to discharge and worsen the stings. Experts recommend using a forceful shower of salt water to remove the microscopic stinging cells; a gentle shower is more likely to cause the cells to discharge, worsening the stings. A cold pack may diminish pain, but wipe off any surface moisture before applying it. Some Australians also use hot but not scalding water applied to the sting site, or hot-water immersion for the Australian species of Portuguese man-of-war. The hot-water treatment for jellyfish stings in North America has not been proved so should not be assumed to be effective. Remember, application of cool fresh water worsens certain stings.

Apply soaks of vinegar or rubbing alcohol for thirty minutes or until pain is relieved. Baking soda powder or paste is recommended to detoxify the sting of certain sea nettles, such as the Chesapeake Bay sea nettle. If these decontaminants are not available, apply soaks of diluted (quarter-strength) household ammonia. A paste made from unseasoned meat tenderizer (do not exceed fifteen minutes of application time, particularly on the sensitive skin of small children) or papaya fruit may be helpful. These contain papain, which may alleviate the sting from the thimble jellyfish that causes seabather's eruption. Do not apply any organic solvent, such as kerosene, turpentine, or gasoline. While likely not harmful, urine has never been proved to be effective.

After decontamination, apply a lather of shaving cream or soap and shave the affected area with a razor. In a pinch, you can use a paste of sand or mud in seawater and a clamshell.

Reapply the vinegar or rubbing alcohol soak for fifteen minutes.

Apply a thin coating of hydrocortisone lotion (0.5 to 1 percent) twice a day. Anesthetic ointment (such as lidocaine hydrochloride 2.5 percent, or a benzocaine-containing spray) may provide short-term pain relief.

If the victim has a large area involved (an entire arm or leg, face, or genitals), is very young or very old, or shows signs of generalized illness (nausea, vomiting, weakness, shortness of breath, or chest pain), seek help from a doctor. If a child has placed tentacle fragments in his mouth, have him swish and spit whatever potable liquid is available. If there is already swelling in the mouth (muffled voice, difficulty swallowing, enlarged tongue and lips), do not give anything by mouth, protect the airway, and rapidly transport the victim to a hospital. Note: Protecting the airway is done by intubating the victim. Anaphylaxis can set in (quickly), and once the airway is swollen shut, you cannot get it open unless you cut (cricotomy). A jellyfish sting in the mouth is dangerous due to the swelling in the airway. ABCs (airway, breathing, circulation) must be monitored quickly. The EMT/paramedic may forgo any risks and intubate, even if the patient is conscious.

Treatment for Hawaii Man-of-War Species

Rinse the area liberally with seawater or fresh water to remove any tentacles stuck to the skin. This can be from a spray bottle or in a beach shower. Do not apply vinegar.

For severe pain, try applying heat or cold—whichever feels better to the victim.

Few Portuguese man-of-war stings in Hawaii cause a life-threatening reaction, but it is always a possibility. Some people are extremely sensitive to the venom; a few have allergic reactions. You should consider even the slightest difficulty breathing, or altered level of consciousness, to be a medical emergency. If a severe allergic reaction is suspected or diagnosed, call for help and use an automatic epinephrine injector, if available, and if someone is qualified to administer the injection.

This differs from the advice offered by Dr. Auerbach. Some of the lifeguards cite a study showing that vinegar sometimes makes the sting worse. Portuguese man-of-wars belong to a different family than box jellyfish [Carybdea alata] and therefore must be treated separately. It is a personal choice whether or not to use vinegar to treat Pacific man-of-war stings.

LEPTOSPIROSIS

Leptospirosis is caused by the *Leptospira spirochete*. It's a problem worldwide in bodies of fresh and salt water. Leptospirosis can be carried by many animals, such as rats, skunks, opossums, raccoons, foxes, and other vermin. It is transmitted when people come in contact with infected soil or water (contaminated with the waste products of an infected animal). People contract the disease by either eating contaminated food or water or through cuts and via the eyes, nose, and mouth if they come in contact with the contaminated water or soil.

Leptospirosis occurs in fresh and salt water all over the world, but it is most common in the tropics. The U.S. Centers for Disease Control and Prevention states that there are between one and two hundred cases of leptospirosis reported each year in the United States, with about 50 percent of cases occurring in Hawaii.

Medical experts describe flulike symptoms, headaches, muscle aches, eye pain, and red eyes, followed by chills and fever. By the fifth or sixth day, the second phase of the illness begins, with fever and aching, stiffness of the neck, and serious inflammation of the nerves to the eyes, brain, spinal column, and other structures. Right upper-quadrant abdominal pain may occur.

Dr. Laura King said that:

~ The treatment of non-severe cases is with oral doxycycline or tetracycline.
~ The treatment for serious cases is intravenous penicillin G or third-generation cephalosporins.

SEABATHER'S ERUPTION

Seabather's eruption on the skin is caused by stinging cells from the thimble jellyfish, such as *Linuche unguiculata*, and the larval forms of certain sea anemones, such as *Edwardsiella lineata*. Swimmers may feel tingling sensations on exposed skin or beneath a swimsuit while they are swimming. The stings from these tiny sea animals cause a rash accompanied by intense itching and pain. Dr. Auerbach noted that most first remedies are not very satisfying.

Vinegar or rubbing alcohol can be used, but neither is very effective. Unseasoned meat tenderizer (papain) may help the initial decontamination, followed by an application of calamine lotion to soothe the skin. The swimmer should treat the skin with a topical decontaminant before taking a bath or shower; otherwise, the fresh water will likely make the reaction worse. After decontaminating and thoroughly washing your skin with soap and water, try applying a topical steroid preparation.

The sting cells remain within the swimsuit and continue to cause a problem, so the swimsuit needs to be washed in a machine on a full cycle or rinsed with vinegar or alcohol and then washed with soap and water, taking care to wear rubber dishwashing gloves.

To prevent seabather's eruption, you may want to wear the stinger suit that many Australians use, or a dive skin, but don't overheat and be sure to keep up with your hydration needs. If you wear a garment in the water, prevent chafing by applying a lubricant such as Vaseline, Aquaphor, or BodyGlide. Safe Sea may help block seabather's eruption and is available with or without sun block. Because any topical preparation washes off in the water, reapply it according to the manufacturer's instructions.

SEA CUCUMBERS

Sea cucumbers are cucumber-shaped sea animals that may produce a liquid called holothurin, which causes skin and eye irritation. They range in size from half an inch up to sixteen feet. They look like they would be soft, but their top skin covers many microscopic pieces of skeleton called spicules. Most sea cucumbers live on the sea floor or dig themselves into soft mud or sand. They also live in underwater rock crevices and on the underside of stones and boulders and some sea cucumbers can swim.

It is simply best not to handle them. If swimmers get holothurin in their eyes, Dr. Auerbach recommends irrigating the eyes with at least a quart of disinfected water and seeking immediate medical attention. If the victim is out at sea, treat the eye injury as a corneal abrasion—by instilling ophthalmic antibiotic drops or ointment.

SEA URCHIN

Sea urchins are round-to-flattened bodies with hard shells covered with spines ranging from approximately half an inch to many inches long. The spines serve as protection from predators such as sea otters, wolf eels, and other fish. Sea urchins inhabit all the world's oceans and live in shallow sandy water, rocky areas, and around kelp beds. They vary in size from one and a half inches to about four inches and resemble pincushions, some with short spines (merely an inch long), others with sharp spines over three inches long. They are often green, black, purple, brown, red, and light orange.

Divers hunt for sea urchins for their roe. They usually find them moving slowly with their articulating spines and on tubed feet as they feed on algae and detritus. When you're swimming above, they are beautiful to watch; if their spines are long, they move in the direction of the underwater current. Sea urchins are a favorite food of wolf eel, triggerfish, and sea otters.

The problem is when people mishandle or step on them. The urchin spines that are sharp usually contain venom and can puncture or break beneath the skin. Some types of urchins can grasp the swimmer with small appendages called pedicellaria, which are also venom bearing. Any envenomation can cause severe pain, muscle spasm, or in the case of multiple punctures, difficulty breathing, weakness, low blood pressure, and collapse.

Most commonly, spines become embedded and cause problems as foreign bodies within the soft tissues, leading to inflammation, occasional infection, and complications, such as nerve irritation or arthritis.

Sea Urchin Treatment

Dr. Auerbach and other medical experts recommend the following treatment:

If the injured person is having difficulty breathing and suffering from tightness in the chest, he should go immediately to an emergency department or other qualified medical facility. Otherwise, immerse the wound in nonscalding hot water to tolerance (see the recommendations for scorpion fish, below) for thirty to ninety minutes. Maintain the water temperature by adding more hot water as needed. The hot-water treatment usually reduces pain. Take pain medications as appropriate.

Carefully use tweezers and remove easily extracted visible spines. Do not dig in to the soft tissues, which may cause the spines to become fragmented and make them more difficult to remove. If you see purple or black markings in the skin immediately after it has been penetrated by the spines, that does not always indicate there are spines retained in the skin. The discoloration may be caused by pigment that has leached from the spine(s) into the tissues. The dye will usually be absorbed over a day or two, and the discoloration will then disappear. If there are still black markings after forty-eight to seventy-two hours, a spine fragment is likely present.

If the sting is caused by a species of sea urchin with pincer organs, remove the pedicellaria—the urchins' seizing organs between the spines—by applying shaving cream or a paste of soap and then shaving the affected area, gently scraping with the razor. Scrub the puncture area with soap and water, and flush repeatedly with disinfected fresh water. Treat the wounds with a very light application of antiseptic ointment and dressing.

If the spines are in swimmers' hands or feet, or near joints, they may need to be removed surgically to reduce infection, inflammation, and possible damage to nerves or important blood vessels.

If the wound shows signs of infection (increasing redness, fever, pus, and/or swollen lymph glands within twenty-four to forty-eight hours after the injury) or if the spine is felt to have penetrated into a joint, a physician may want to start the victim on an antibiotic to oppose Vibrio bacteria. Suggested antibiotics are ciprofloxacin, sulfamethoxazole/trimethoprim, doxycycline, or tetracycline, as well as an antibiotic to oppose Staphylococcus bacteria (for example, dicloxacillin or cephalexin).

If a spine puncture in the palm of the hand results in a persistent swollen finger without any sign of infection—namely, fever, redness, or swollen lymph glands in the elbow or armpit—it may be necessary to seek medical treatment. It is possible that there is a retained spine or fragments that have inflamed a tendon, ligament, or soft tissue.

SEAWEED DERMATITIS

Off the shores of Hawaii and Florida is a blue-green algae, *Microcoleus lyngbyaceus*, that slips inside swimsuits. The algae irritates the skin, making it red and itchy, and sometimes it blisters. This reaction may occur just after the swimmer leaves the water.

~ Remove your swimsuit, scrub the skin with soap and water, and rinse with rubbing alcohol.
~ If the reaction is severe, consult a physician.
~ Wash the swimsuit thoroughly.

SCORPION FISH

It's simple—don't touch scorpion fish, and watch where you step. Scorpaenidae, the scorpion fish, is a fish family that includes: zebra fish, lionfish, turkey fish, and scorpion fish. They live in the tropical and temperate seas and are found in the Red Sea, the Caribbean Sea, and the Indo-Pacific Ocean. Shared features of the scorpion fish family are: highly compressed body, large mouth, spines on the head, the gills, and the dorsal and pectoral fins, and they can camouflage themselves by changing colors to match their environment. Sometimes they resemble pieces of coral or rock. Changing colors helps them hunt prey and defend themselves. They usually inhabit the shallow waters, but some species reside at a depth of 7,200 feet. They are solitary in nature and live in caves, crevices, and among the coral reefs.

Scorpion fish have dorsal, anal, and pelvic spines that transport venom from glands into puncture wounds. If a person is stung by a scorpion fish, depending on the species, the wound may be extremely painful, swollen, pale, blistered, or discolored, and accompanied by abdominal pain, shortness of breath, and more severe systemic symptoms. A sting from a scorpion fish may be life threatening.

The treatment for a scorpion fish sting is to immerse the injured area in water as hot as the person can tolerate for thirty to ninety minutes, taking care not to cause a scald injury; always test the hot water on an uninjured part of the body first. The hot water will decrease the swimmer's pain substantially if the sting was from a lionfish. It will have less effect on a scorpion fish sting and little effect on a stonefish sting. Whether or not the pain is diminished, the immersion treatment should be performed, because the heat may decrease the effects of the harmful proteins contained in the venom. Dr. Auerbach noted:

~ Seek immediate medical attention if the victim appears intoxicated or is weak, vomiting, short of breath, or unconscious.
~ It may be necessary for a physician to treat not only the wound but any ensuing infection.
~ There is now antivenom for stonefish. If stung by a stonefish, seek immediate medical attention.

CROWN-OF-THORNS STARFISH

Starfish, or sea stars, are echinoderms, and they belong to the class Asteroidea.

There are about eighteen hundred species of starfish that occur in the world's oceans, including the Atlantic, Pacific, Indian, Arctic, and Southern Ocean Antarctic regions. They live at a range of depths, from the intertidal waters down to abyssal depths of up to six thousand meters. The species vary greatly in size, color, and shape: from the pink starfish to the bright blue starfish and the bat starfish, whose appendages are shaped like bat wings.

The starfish that poses a threat to the environment and swimmers is the crown-of-thorns starfish (*Acanthaster planci*). They are predators of coral reefs. An individual starfish can consume up to sixty-five square feet of living coral reef per year. They are beautiful vibrant-colored starfish with sharp spines on their appendages, up to three inches long, that give them a crownlike shape. They measure about ten inches and are found in tropical oceans around the world. They are dangerous to humans; do not touch them.

The crown-of-thorns starfish produces a neurotoxin that is released through its sharp spines and can easily puncture wet suits and divers' gloves. Wounds from the starfish can be serious, and the neurotoxin can cause a sharp stinging pain that may last for hours, as well as nausea, vomiting, brief muscle paralysis, and swollen glands. The area around the wound often turns dark blue and begins to swell. The swelling may continue for many weeks.

The treatment is similar to that for a sea urchin puncture: Immerse the wound in nonscalding hot water, as hot as the swimmer can tolerate, for thirty to ninety minutes. This frequently provides pain relief.

~ The swimmer may want to take appropriate over-the-counter pain medicine, like ibuprofen.
~ Carefully remove any spines with tweezers.
~ If spines or fragments of spines remain in the wound, seek the assistance of a physician.

STONEFISH

The Australian Aborigines perform an ancient dance in which a man wades into a tidal pool to hunt for fish. He suddenly steps on something and screams from the pain. The dancer writhes on the ground, and the dance ends with a death song. The stonefish dance is meant to educate the young Aborigines about the dangers of stonefish, the deadliest fish in the world.

Stonefish, a genus of fish of the family Synanceiidae, inhabit the Indo-Pacific and northern Australian waters and grow to be up to twelve inches long. They are found in exposed sand and mud tidal inlets to depths of about 120 feet. They are mottled brownish green and perfectly camouflaged to look like kelp-covered rocks. When disturbed or threatened, they stick up their thirteen dorsal spines, and glands along their back project venom into the spines. Stonefish are armed this way against predatory sharks and rays, but they also present great danger to swimmers.

The stonefish sting causes excruciating pain, rapid swelling, and tissue death. The severity of the sting and symptoms depends on the depth of penetration and the number of spines involved. The venom can cause muscle weakness, temporary paralysis, and shock, which may result in death if not treated. Fatalities have occurred in the Indo-Pacific region, though not in Australian waters.

If stung:

~ Bathing or immersing the sting in hot water may reduce the pain.
~ Transport the patient to the nearest hospital.

STINGRAYS

Stingrays are found in coastal tropical and subtropical marine waters throughout the world, and there are some species that inhabit temperate oceans, deep oceans, and rivers. Stingrays are a group of rays that are cartilaginous fish related to sharks. Most stingrays have one or multiple barbed stingers on their tails. The barb is about two inches long, and its underside has two grooves with venom glands. The stinger is covered with a thin layer of skin, the integumentary sheath, in which the venom is concentrated. Stingrays do not aggressively attack humans; usually, stings occur only if a ray is accidentally stepped on. To avoid stepping on a stingray, lifeguards advise shuffling your feet when you are entering and exiting the water.

If you're stung, seek assistance from a beach lifeguard. If you begin to feel tightness in the chest, swelling anywhere on your face, difficulty breathing, hives anywhere on your body, or nausea, you are having an allergic reaction! Get to an emergency room immediately! Allergic reactions can be minor to severe, so any abnormal reactions besides occasional itching, minor swelling at the sting site, or pain should be seen by a doctor.

~ If in doubt, always seek medical attention, especially if the wound becomes inflamed or infection does not subside after a few days of at-home treatment.

~ People with compromised immune systems need to seek immediate medical treatment.

~ Place the area that was stung in a bucket of very hot water to denature (break down the stingray venom).

~ After the pain has diminished, use topical antibiotics such as Neosporin or Bactine.

~ The wound may be bandaged. Make sure it does not reduce circulation to the area.

~ Check the wound for infection.

COUNTRY MEDICINE

Years ago, Don Nelson, a marine biologist from California State University, Long Beach, told me that meat tenderizer was an effective treatment for jellyfish stings. It has a papaya enzyme that breaks down the protein of nematocyst, the stinging cell that that jellyfish inject into skin when a swimmer brushes against the tentacles.

The origin for this wisdom may have come from the people living in Micronesia. Cindy Hunter, my biologist friend who conducts research on coral reefs, was diving off some of the Micronesian Islands, where there are many species of jellyfish. The local people told her that when they were stung, they placed papaya skins on the sting sites.

Recently, two friends, Sandy and Janice, were doing a training swim off Corona del Mar, California. Janice was stung. Sandy had some meat tenderizer in her car and rubbed it on Janice's wound, then gave her a couple of Advils while they waited for the lifeguards to transport her to the lifeguard station. By the time they immersed her foot in hot water, the meat tenderizer had done its job, and the pain had pretty much disappeared.

Dr. Auerbach added, "One must take care to not leave meat tenderizer on sensitive skin for too long, no longer than ten to fifteen minutes, because it can cause an irritating reaction in and of itself. Furthermore, I have heard from a few users that if the seasoned form of tenderizer is used, it may increase the irritation or even cause stinging. The sensitive skin of infants and babies, and facial skin at all ages, may be more prone to an adverse skin irritation from application of papain. I have heard of using fresh papaya fruit. I don't know anything about the use of pineapple."

SWIMMER'S ITCH

Swimmer's itch (also known as duck itch, lake itch, cercarial dermatitis, and Schistosome cercarial dermatitis) is a short-term immune response that happens when a swimmer's skin has been infected by a waterborne flatworm called schistosomatidae. These parasites live in fresh water and salt water and use freshwater snails or waterfowl as their hosts (that may be the origin of the term "duck itch").

Swimmer's itch occurs when the flatworm releases microscopic cercariae into the water and they penetrate the swimmer's skin. The cercariae immediately die and cause an immune reaction beginning as mild itchy spots that may worsen. This occurs mostly in summer and was diagnosed first in Lake Michigan.

The symptoms are itchy raised papules within a few hours of the infection, but they are usually gone within a week. I wish I'd known before I began training in Lake Titicaca, Bolivia. After my first day of training, I broke out all over my body in pink welts about the size of quarters. They itched mildly at first, and then the itching intensified. I was driving Pete Kelly, my crew member, nuts with my scratching. Pete, who spoke fluent Spanish, tried his best to find out what was causing the welts. On the street in Copacabana, he stopped a local woman and showed her the bumps on my neck. She gave us a horrified look, quickly made the sign of the cross, and turned and ran away, as if I had bubonic plague.

Not to be deterred, Pete continued his search and found a local pharmacist who told him that in the jungles of South America, the native Indians used something called violetta, the juice from the fruit of an indigenous plant, to stop the itch of mosquito bites. Pete thought violetta might help me stop itching.

The pharmacist had some on hand in a small bottle, and I applied the solution liberally to the welts. It turned them deep purple but did not do anything to diminish the itch. Pete encouraged me to continue applying it, for lack of anything better to do. Soon my body was covered by itchy pink and purple polka dots. And red polka dots where the dots blistered. In a week, they went away on their own.

We never noticed any freshwater snails in the water or waterfowl swimming around the lake, just small groups of brown and white cows that stood like statues, ankle-deep in the water, and slowly turned their heads from left to right and back as I swam past.

When I arrived home and Dr. King noticed the welts on my skin, she said I probably had swimmer's itch. It was a relief to know that it wasn't a strange disease, and it helped to know how to treat it. Most people think that swimmer's itch only occurs in freshwater lakes, but Dr. King says it can happen in salt water, too. Dr. King and Dr. Auerbach recommend the following treatment: Rinse the skin with rubbing alcohol and coat it with calamine or Caladryl lotion. Additional treatments include baking soda or oatmeal baths. Topical steroid creams help reduce the itching. If the reaction is severe, you should see a physician. Cercariae are found in greatest concentrations in warm shallow waters and in areas where there are long grasses that serve as home to the snails. Simply avoid swimming in these areas.

SEALS RECOMMEND *U.S. NAVY DIVE MANUAL*

Above are some of the more dangerous marine animals that swimmers may encounter, but there are many other dangerous marine animals, and it is worth thoroughly researching any area before you swim.

The SEALs use the *U.S. Navy Dive Manual*, which can be downloaded for free from the Internet (see Sources for website address; page 301). They recommend Revision 6, volume 5, appendices 5B and 5C, which cover diving first aid and dangerous marine life, respectively.

Chapter 14

Sharks

A friend once suggested that I attempt a swim across Lake Nicaragua. He explained that it was the largest lake in Central America, bordered by the Pacific Ocean on the west and the Caribbean Sea on the east and connected by the San Juan River to the Caribbean Sea. It sounded interesting, and all the tourist brochures touted great tarpon fishing, which made me think that it would be fairly easy to find an escort boat for the swim.

When I mentioned the idea to Laura, my sister who coached at Alamo Area Aquatic Association in San Antonio, Texas, she said she would check with Solomon Soza, a friend who coached with her and had grown up in Central America.

Solomon had seen tourist brochures about Lake Nicaragua or, as it was known in Spanish, Mar Dulce ("The Sweet Sea"). Brochures touted the beauty of the lake, but after he checked with friends who had been to the area, he discovered that Lake Nicaragua was anything but fresh; it was seriously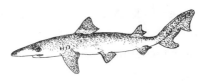

polluted by sewage. In 1981 thirty-two tons (seventy thousand pounds) of raw sewage was being released into Lake Nicaragua daily, and the industries along the shore had been dumping chemicals and other pollutants in it for a long time.

More than that, Solomon said that there was a large population of sharks living in the lake. My first thought was that Solomon was joking; I had never heard of freshwater sharks. I checked with another friend, Bob Gelbard, who had been the assistant secretary of state for Latin America, and was a swimmer and diver. Bob confirmed that there were bull sharks in Lake Nicaragua and it was dangerous to swim there. People had been attacked by the sharks and also by sawfish. Bob explained that sawfish live in tropical and subtropical areas in the Atlantic and Indo-Pacific, in coastal waters, estuaries, bays, rivers, and lakes. They inhabit shallow murky waters and can move back and forth between salt and fresh water. Sawfish are usually light gray or brown and are related to sharks and rays, though they have more of a shark-shaped body, with a very long snout called a rostrum. The rostrum has sharp "teeth" called denticles, and the sawfish uses it like a saw.

The rostrum is equipped with electroreceptor and motion sensors that can sense the heartbeats and movements of prawns, crabs, and other fish hiding in the mud. They rake the mud with their rostrum to uncover prey hiding in mud, and they use it to slash fast-swimming prey. The species that inhabits Lake Nicaragua, the largetooth sawfish, can grow up to twenty feet long and weigh up to one thousand pounds. They sleep during the day and fish at night. They are not known to attack humans unless provoked or surprised.

I did not want to give up on the idea of swimming across Lake Nicaragua. I thought there might be areas of the lake where the water was not as polluted, and a way to avoid annoying the sawfish. I checked with my friend

Don Nelson, the researcher at California State University, Long Beach. He confirmed that the bull sharks in Lake Nicaragua were especially interesting because they were able to jump over the rapids of the San Juan River and swim between Lake Nicaragua and the Caribbean Sea. He noted that bull sharks were particularly aggressive, and he did not advise swimming in the lake.

Don knew about aggressive sharks. He had spent much of his career studying gray reef sharks in Tahiti and around Enewetak Atol with Richard Johnson, another shark expert. The reef sharks were between four and five feet long. Don said they noticed that if they swam too close to a gray reef shark or if they made fast, startling movements, the shark would swim in an exaggerated manner, wagging its head and tail from side to side. It would point its pectoral fins (the fins on the underside of its body) downward, lift its snout, arch its back, and sometimes swim in a rolling or spiraling motion. Don said that if a shark was cornered, its behavior became more aggressive, though this was not unusual behavior for any cornered animal.

Don said he got too close to one four- or five-foot-long shark, and it bit his arm. Don's eyes lit up when he talked about the speed with which the shark struck. Fortunately, he was wearing Kevlar for protection, so he wasn't badly hurt. The experience didn't dampen his fascination with sharks.

When I would call and tell him that I was thinking about swimming in a certain waterway, he'd open his encyclopedia that showed the waterways of the world, and the species of sharks that inhabited them, and describe in wonderful detail the species in the waters, how big they grew, and how they behaved. He told me about all species of sharks, including pygmy sharks that were eight to ten inches in length, with photophores that produced bioluminescent light on their undersides. The photophores were used for protective "counter shading" camouflage, to make them less visible against the lighter background at the surface.

One of my favorites was the Wobbegong shark, a three- or four-foot-long shark that lives in the shallow waters off Australia. Their bodies are camouflaged with a symmetrical pattern of bold markings that resemble a carpet, so Wobbegongs are often known as carpet sharks. The small whisker lobes surrounding the jaw are used to attract and catch fish. They are relatively invisible around rocky shores. They don't attack swimmers or divers but will bite if harassed or stepped on.

Don's enthusiasm for sharks was contagious. He said that of the 360 species of sharks, only four—the great white, oceanic whitetip, tiger, and bull sharks—are threatening to humans. Although all four are large, powerful predators known to have attacked and killed people, they have been filmed without the photographer using a cage for protection.

Once when I was speaking, I met a woman at the University of Hawaii who loved swimming in the open water. Sharks were her family's aumakua. She explained that aumakua are deified ancestor guardians that watch over members of a native Hawaiian's clan. Different clans have different animals. Sharks are the most popular aumakua, but sea turtles are as well.

Because sharks were her family's guardians, she always felt safe when she swam offshore. She mentioned that she and her brother went fishing one time off Oahu. They had been out five hours, and the tropical sun was very hot, so she told her brother to stop fishing. She wanted to jump into the water and swim.

Within minutes her brother saw a large shark fin moving toward her. He thought it was a tiger shark, maybe twelve feet long. He shouted and tried to move the boat to her before the shark got too close. But there wasn't time.

She saw the shark swimming toward her and around her, but she was not afraid. She talked to the shark, and it eventually swam away. She knew of members of her clan who kept a hammerhead shark as a pet. They fed it and petted it like a dog. Having a shark as a pet was part of her clan's tradition.

Who knows what sharks sense and how bonds are created between sharks and humans. This was something new to me but not to Eugenie Clark, a renowned expert in shark research who developed one of the first shark repellents from a fish called the Moses sole. The Moses sole emits a substance that has the same chemistry as soap. Eugenie tied the Moses sole with a string and lowered it into the water, and the sharks swam toward the sole, then turned away. They ate other species of fish, but the Moses sole always remained untouched. Don Nelson said it was a promising repellent, but in order for it to work, you had to squirt the substance the shark's mouth. Sharks didn't like their mouths washed out with soap.

Before going snorkeling in the Caribbean, I asked Eugenie Clark for advice. "It's a rare opportunity to see sharks. When else could you observe sharks in the wild?" Maybe if I observed them in their natural surroundings, I thought, I would understand them better and be less afraid. The divemaster off Walker's Cay tossed frozen bait into the water. It sank to the shallow ocean floor. With one of the crew members, I jumped in the water to watch Caribbean reef sharks, four to five feet long, swim in and feed off the chum. They were fairly shy and stayed at least ten feet away. A seven- or eight-foot bull shark swam right below us, focusing on the chum but only three feet away. I kept hearing Don Nelson's voice in my head: "Bull sharks can be very dangerous. You want to avoid bull sharks."

Other sharks swam in to feed off the chum, and another bull shark, this one six or seven feet, joined the dinner party. It was amazing to watch them swim and feed, and I did gain a greater appreciation of them, but I never felt comfortable.

Don gave me some general guidelines about swimming anywhere in the ocean:

~ Before swimming in any waterway, check with the local beach lifeguard, coast guard, divemasters, or harbormaster to find out if there is a shark problem.

~ Don't wear a swimsuit lined with metallic material or wear jewelry. Shiny metal attracts attention from sharks and barracuda.

~ In areas where there are seals and sea lions, don't wear black swimsuits. These animals are the primary food source for great white sharks, and it is not good to resemble food.

~ Seals, sea lions, elephant seals, and sea turtles are the primary food source for some large sharks, such as great whites. It is not good to swim in a feeding area. Avoid rookeries or places where there are high concentrations of these marine mammals. A swimmer could be mistaken for food.

~ "When in doubt, get out" is my motto. If you are swimming in an area in which you don't feel comfortable, get out of the water.

According to John McCosker, formerly the director of the Steinhart Aquarium and currently the senior scientist and chair of the California Academy of Sciences in San Francisco, "The danger of shark attack in California waters is minuscule; however, should one have that experience, it can be a very serious and most unforgettable event. Only ninety-nine unprovoked attacks by sharks (all or nearly all involving the white shark, *Carcharodon carcharias*), resulting in nine fatalities, have occurred in California history. An average of 1.8 attacks per year have occurred in California during the last decade, which is far fewer than the numerous drownings, bee stings, and lightning strikes that cause fatalities each year."

SWIMMING WITH SHARKS AND RAYS

Christopher Lowe, PhD, is a professor in the Department of Biological Sciences at California State University, Long Beach, and at one point during his career, he studied with Don Nelson. Dr. Lowe is one of the world's foremost experts on sharks. He grew up on Martha's Vineyard and spent hours swimming and fishing offshore. His favorite catch was sharks. He said that they come in so many different shapes and sizes that it is hard to sum them up in a single description. He said, "The lovable horn shark always reminds me of a puppy. They have large pectoral fins, big old horned dorsal fins, and that funny punched-in nose. Watching them eat sea urchins always cracks me up. It's like watching a puppy trying to eat a bug for the first time. Not many people would use the word 'cute' and 'shark' in the same sentence, but how can you not when you see a horn shark? And the regal silvertip shark is by far one of my favorite tropical reef sharks. With their sleek lines and dapper silver-tipped fins, they epitomize poise and grace. Having worked with some many species over the years, I find it interesting how each species has a unique personality. They are all amazingly strong and can move incredibly fast when needed."

While many people dread the thought of swimming with sharks, Dr. Lowe seeks them out. He said, "I've had the wonderful opportunity to swim and dive with a lot of different species of sharks. Most of the encounters were intentional—I was out looking for them. I can remember seeing a large tiger shark in the water at Midway Atoll and swimming as hard as I could to take a picture of it, but it leisurely swam away from me, leaving me behind with the plankton! I've never seen a white shark while swimming or diving. With all the time I've spent in the water off California, I'm certain a few have cruised by me and I didn't even know it. But that is the predator's gift—the ability to see without being seen. It doesn't really worry me to be in the water with sharks, though I do try to be observant and aware. Situational awareness is a very useful sense when you're in the water. A good predator knows when they're being spotted, and the jig is up. If you watch fish around sharks, they are always keeping their eyes on them and moving in ways to maintain vigilance. Usually, under these circumstances, the shark either moves on or changes its behavior."

Many swimmers are concerned that swimming motions could attract sharks, but Dr. Lowe said, "While the splashing created by a swimmer is easily detected by a shark, the constant rhythm of splashing from a swimmer is probably very different than that of a seal or sea turtle. Seals are also good predators, and a lot of splashing will give them away, so it would be unlikely for a seal or sea turtle to produce a rhythmic splashing sound like a swimmer. Scuba divers are a good example of a foreign, noisy critter in the water. Most of the noise comes from the regulator. Most sharks seem to avoid scuba divers that use open circuit systems and exhale noisy bubbles; however, the increased popularity of rebreathers indicates that the quieter systems are not as off-putting to sharks. As a result, some scientists have suggested using some sort of device that produces an unusual mechanical noise—a kind of cowbell for bears."

Dr. Lowe said, "I think the best thing a swimmer can do is to be aware and observant. You won't walk through a 'bad' neighborhood at night without a buddy or while wearing headphones and reading a book. Most predators lose interest if they know that their potential prey is aware of their presence and ready to respond. It takes away their advantage. So, don't make yourself a target; look alert while you swim. Obviously, some areas have higher shark populations than others, so it is always good to do your homework before you swim in an area, and find out what kinds of marine life are common there. Swimming in central and northern California in late summer and fall is not prudent due to the number of white sharks in coastal waters then. You are much more likely to encounter sharks on ocean swims in tropical waters than temperate waters; however, a lot depends on the region. A quick Google search will turn up a lot about sharks in your area."

There is a huge concern about the decline of shark populations, which is upsetting the natural balance of the oceans. Dr. Lowe said, "Many shark populations have been reduced due to overfishing. The reef sharks are the most susceptible due to their more limited wanderings, but even nomadic oceanic species have been impacted. We really don't understand how pollution affects sharks, but we do know that many species accumulate large concentrations of mercury and other contaminants through the food web. Based on our understanding of how these contaminants affect mammals, it is likely they pose health threats to sharks as well. There is some good news, though; better fisheries management and cleaner water in some regions, such as California, are allowing shark populations to recover. If we all work together, future generations may be able to see sharks when they're out for a nice swim!"

MINDS IN THE WATER

A few years ago, Bob West, the "kingpin" of the La Jolla group that swims in La Jolla Cove, invited Oliver Sacks and me to swim with him. Bob spent a lot of his life coaching football and swimming in the cove and Oliver grew up swimming in the sea off the shores of England. Bob couldn't wait to take us on a coastal tour. He promised we would see leopard sharks ranging in size from three to four feet; he said he and his pals swam with them all the time. Oliver and I were excited and, I think, a little nervous. Oliver is one of the world's top neurologists, and he writes about people and the dramatic and often beautiful accommodations they make to changes in the way their minds function. Oliver wrote *Awakenings*, *The Man Who Mistook His Wife for a Hat*, *Musicophillia*, and many other books. He was in his early seventies and swimming and writing and going strong.

We slipped under the waves and swam toward the buoy line that extends from La Jolla Cove to La Jolla Shores. The water was clear, filled with thick kelp that danced with the surf. There were bright orange garibaldi swimming among small rocks and boulders, and spiny sea urchins, and sea bass.

When I turned to breathe, I glanced at Oliver, swimming between Bob and me. His arm strokes looked smooth and effortless, and I could see them both grinning like kids on a new adventure. I smiled and looked at the ocean beyond them and suddenly saw a very large fin sticking out of the water. It was dark and way too big to be a leopard shark's. I stared at it to make sure I wasn't mistaken and then saw a second, larger fin right beside the first. The fins weren't moving from side to side, the way a shark's would, but I wondered if I should say something. A swell lifted the fins high above the water, and I saw the two animals attached to them. They were seals. I started laughing. Bob and Oliver saw me and stopped, and I pointed toward the seals and said, "Looks like a Gary Larson cartoon. The seals have their flippers above their heads like they're imitating great white sharks!"

Bob explained that seals often rest on the water that way, and wondered if they were extending their flippers to warm them in the sun. When we swam by a rocky outcropping, I noticed a group of California sea lions resting on the rocks with their hind flippers lifted toward the sun. I held my breath as we swam past the rocks. The seals exuded a strong smell of excrement.

We continued toward La Jolla Shores and swam above three leopard sharks hiding in screens of kelp. Their beautiful bodies were covered with black saddle-like markings and large spots on their backs. They turned slightly and then swam right beneath Oliver. They seemed to slow and watch him, and I told him that with all the freckles he had on his shoulders, the leopard sharks probably thought he was their cousin.

A few years later, when I was corresponding with L. Tadeus and trying to find better ways to rewarm after cold exposure, the SEAL officer told me about a heating/cooling device being developed at Stanford University by Dennis Grahn, PhD, and Chuck Hixson, with a company called AVAcore. They are working with the U.S. military to test this device. The idea is to have a hypothermic/hyperthermic person place a hand or foot in the device, which will warm or cool the hand or foot and, in turn, heat or cool the person's core. Perhaps the sea lions knew innately how to warm their core by extending their flippers.

While it was fascinating to swim with sharks and sea lions in La Jolla Cove, it is not something I would ordinarily do. I realize that I am taking on more risk because they are wild animals; they are unpredictable and can be aggressive. A couple of years ago, fourteen swimmers who routinely swam in the bay over a few weeks' time were bitten by a California sea lion. Wildlife experts thought that swimmers may have swum too close to a rookery during breeding season, or the sea lion may have eaten shellfish and sardines that had fed on phytoplankton, thereby producing domoic acid, and the sea lion became sick and aggressive when the toxins affected his brain.

U.S. NAVY DIVING MANUAL ON SHARKS

While shark attacks are uncommon, it's important to know what to do if one occurs. According to the *U.S. Navy Diving Manual*, there have been only forty to one hundred shark attacks since 1965. The shark attacks were unpredictable and the injuries were caused by bites and by coming in contact with the shark's skin. Sharkskin is incredibly rough and covered with sharp dentine appendages called denticles. Rubbing against them can cause severe bleeding.

There are certain pre-attack behaviors that are predictable. According to the *Manual*, "A shark preparing to attack swims with an exaggerated motion, its pectoral fins pointing down in contrast to the usual flared-out position, and it swims in circles of decreasing radius around the prey. An attack may be heralded by unexpected acceleration or other marked change in behavior, posture, or swim patterns. Should surrounding schools of fish become unexplainably agitated, sharks may be in the area. Sharks are much faster and more powerful than any swimmer. All sharks must be treated with extreme respect and caution."

FIRST AID FOR SHARK BITES

Bites may result in a large amount of bleeding and tissue loss. Recommendations from the *U.S. Navy Diving Manual*:

- ~ Get out of the water immediately.
- ~ Take immediate action to control bleeding, using large gauze pressure bandages.
- ~ Cover wounds with layers of compressive dressings, preferably made with gauze but easily made from shirts or towels, and held in place by wrapping the wound tightly with gauze, torn clothing, towels, or sheets.
- ~ Direct pressure with elevation or extreme compression on pressure points will control all but the most serious bleeding. The major pressure points are: the radial artery pulse point for the hand; above the elbow under the biceps muscle for the forearm (brachial artery); and the groin area with deep fingertip or heel-of-the-hand pressure for bleeding from the leg (femoral artery).
- ~ When bleeding cannot be controlled by direct pressure

and elevation or pressure points, a tourniquet or ligature may be needed to save the victim's life, even though there is the possibility of loss of the limb.

~ Tourniquets are applied only as a last resort and with only enough pressure to control bleeding. Do not remove the tourniquet. The tourniquet should be removed only by a physician in a hospital setting. Loosening of a tourniquet may cause further shock by releasing toxins into the circulatory system from the injured limb as well as continued blood loss.

~ Treat for shock by laying the patient down and elevating his feet.

~ If medical personnel are available, begin intravenous (IV) Ringer's lactate or normal saline with a large-bore cannula (16 or 18 gallons). If blood loss has been extensive, several liters should be infused rapidly.

~ The patient's color, pulse, and blood pressure should be used as a guide to the volume of fluid required.

~ Maintain an airway and administer oxygen. Do not give fluids by mouth. If the patient's cardiovascular state is stable, narcotics may be administered in small doses for pain relief. Observe closely for evidence of depressed respirations due to the use of narcotics.

~ Initial stabilization procedures should include attention to the airway, breathing, and circulation, followed by a complete evaluation for multiple trauma.

~ Transport the victim to a medical facility as soon as possible. Reassure the patient.

Remember that shark attacks are rare. The Florida Museum of Natural History's International Shark Attack File states that the United States averages less than one shark-attack death per year (see Sources for website address; page 301). According to Oceana, an international conservation organization focused on protecting and restoring the world's oceans, one hundred million sharks are killed each year by industrial fishing.

PART FOUR

Advanced Swimmers

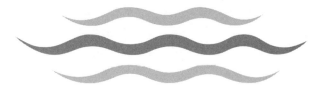

~~~

Chapter 15

Into the Dark

SWIMMING IN THE DARK

When people swim across the Catalina Channel and English Channel, they usually make at least part of the crossing in the dark. When the sun goes down, the wind often dies, so the ocean lies down, and it is much easier to swim across calm seas.

Swimming in the dark is very different from swimming during daylight. It is literally the difference between night and day. Some people are uncomfortable and fearful during dark swims. Other people love being immersed in the dark, swimming through eerie black waters that glow iridescent white and phosphorescent green. They love the silky blackness of smooth curling waters, and they love to watch the night sky and the progression of the moon, stars, and planets.

When a group of swimmers from Seal Beach let me train with them to swim across the Catalina Channel, it was all a grand adventure. We looked forward to what would happen next. Our coach tried to prepare us as well as he could, and he was open-minded. My father suggested that we work out at night. He thought it would help our body clocks adjust, since we would be starting from Catalina Island at midnight, when the wind was down and the seas were calm.

He also thought swimming in the darkness of night and early morning would teach us how to see in the darkness, how to listen more intently for approaching motorboats and the coach's voice. We would have to swim closer together and learn not to bump into one another. We learned to navigate better, how to use the small red and green lights on the distant oil rigs in Long Beach and the amber glowing streetlights that lined the Seal Beach Pier.

At night and during the morning darkness, it was easier to stray off course, because we had fewer visual cues in the dark. It took more focus to find our balance in the water, and more concentration to pull with equal power on our right and left sides so that we stayed on course. It was four or five nights before we were able to consistently swim close together and maintain a straight course, but there were times when we spaced out and hit someone else with an arm and felt the other swimmer jump and sometimes scream and laugh. We had fun. We were doing something so different, having new experiences, and expanding our worlds.

When planning to do a swim at night, make sure you do some training swims in the dark and have qualified support crew. First try swimming in a bay or harbor, where the water is very calm and there is a lot of light on the water from bridges and boats and alongshore from streetlights and cars.

As you gain more confidence, swim in increasingly darker and rougher waters; always have an experienced kayaker or paddler beside you. Boaters are not expecting swimmers in the dark, and sometimes they cross over into designated swimming areas. The kayaker or paddler needs to be alert to this and know how to move out of the way quickly.

The kayaker should feed you periodically to test out the food you plan to use on your big swim. She should paddle at your pace, observe your stroke rate, and know when you are feeling well and when you are dropping pace. It is helpful if the kayaker is encouraging and honest. It is not helpful if the kayaker is negative.

Communication is even more important during dark swims because the support crew may not be able to see your expressions and tell if you're okay.

DARK SWIMS AND ILLUMINATION

When a group of swimmers contacted me for advice about a relay swim across the Gulf of Baja, one of the questions they asked was: Will there be a problem with sharks? They estimated that the six-man relay team would take roughly four or five days to complete the swim. When they told me they were planning to swim at night, I told them what fishermen had taught me: If you are going to have lights on the water, make sure to keep them to a minimum. Lights attract fish. The more lights you use, the more fish you attract, and eventually, you may attract predatory fish. L. Tadeus commented: "Well-resourced swimmers may want to consider night-vision devices and infrared chem lights/spotlights. You can buy cheap versions of these at Cabela's and other hunting places, such as REI.

"You want your crew to use just enough light so that you can see without attracting fish. And you want to make sure that the support crew can see you in the water."

I've discovered that the support boat's running lights usually give enough light for a swimmer to see the boat, along with small waterproof flashlights that float strapped to the kayak or paddleboard or bow of a Zodiac to help make the kayaker or paddler visible. We always carried extra batteries because if the water was cool, the batteries were depleted faster.

Light-colored swimming caps make you visible in the water. I also suggested that the relay members use reflective tape on the swimming caps, but not so much that they would look like a lure.

After giving them this information, I contacted Chris Lowe to ask about shark populations off Baja. Chris said that he didn't think the sharks would be a problem. But when he discovered that the swimmers planned to use green glow sticks in the back of their swimsuits or attached to their caps, Chris advised to use them sparingly. He explained the fishermen off the shores of Mexico used glow sticks in the Gulf of Baja to attract giant squid. He said on a swim in that area, he would be more concerned about being attacked by a giant squid than by a shark.

FINDING BETTER ILLUMINATION

For years, I've been trying to figure out how to help people swim more safely, especially at night. This concern grew when I heard about a Swiss swimmer who was crossing the English Channel and disappeared into a dark wave and was gone. A few days later, his body was recovered off the shores of Belgium. When I talking with Traci Gray, my friend who is a loadmaster for the United States Air Force, she asked, "Why don't you use lasers? We use them all the time for our C-17."

She explained that if the lasers are positioned correctly, a swimmer can see the boat more easily in the dark and also in the fog. While I haven't had the opportunity to try this advice, it sounds very helpful.

Before we did our dark swims off Seal Beach, we checked the weather forecast. If the weather forecast was for fog, we didn't swim. It is easy to become disoriented or lost in the fog, even if you are only a few yards from the beach.

When the air is hot and the water is cool, fog often

develops. There are many places in the United States and around the world where fog is part of the normal weather pattern. Check the weather forecast before you swim. As an additional precaution, you might want to wear a GPS wristwatch or compass to help you get back to shore if you get caught in the fog.

Chapter 16

Seasickness

For centuries people have traveled by boat and ship and been affected by the movement of water. The Chinese discovered that eating the root of the beautiful leafy and flowering ginger plant and drinking tea made from the root would alleviate the mild symptoms of seasickness. Today cruise ships that travel across the Drake Passage, where sea swells routinely rise to over thirty feet, carry a variety of products: cubes of candied ginger, packets of ginger teas, and a variety of over-the-counter seasickness medications. Getting seasick, whether on the boat before your swim or in the water, can be hell.

When you're in rough water, there's no way to escape a boat's rocking, rolling, and spinning. People tolerate movement across the water differently. Some people get seasick just being on a boat in a harbor, while others can endure very rough seas. A few years ago, my friends and I sailed out of Ushuaia, Argentina, to Antarctica on an icebreaker. Before we left port, we were told that when we crossed the Drake Passage, the waves could be up to eighty feet high. The highest waves I'd sailed through were ten to fifteen feet. I hoped we would experience those huge waves and could only imagine how powerful they'd be.

For two and a half days, the ship constantly met seas that were thirty to forty feet high. The waves did not move in rolling sets; their motion was irregular. The icebreaker shimmied, rocked, rolled, jerked to one side and the other, and then abruptly dropped into a trough or shot up into a crest.

The view from the porthole resembled a washing machine on spin cycle. My two cabinmates had taken sea-sickness medications but weren't able to hold down either those or the candied ginger they had eaten to stave off their queasiness. One friend tried the anti-seasickness patch and experienced one of the side effects—paranoia—and when she got some of the medication on her fingers and rubbed her eyes, they dilated and she was miserable.

Having been on boats in rough seas, I knew I wasn't prone to seasickness, but I had never experienced waves so large and wasn't sure if they would affect me. I couldn't afford to lose electrolytes before my swim, and I didn't want to move around the ship and risk tumbling and breaking an arm, so I lay in my bunk and looked out the porthole. One moment the porthole was covered by spin-ning water, and the next moment there was air.

We were okay until a fifty-foot wave hit the ship so hard, it launched us out of our bunks, broke the hinges on our dresser, and the drawers flew across the room, along with luggage and bedding. For a moment we were stunned, then checked on one another, and when we found that we were all okay, we crawled back into our bunks and lay there laughing. It took my friends a few days after the passage to feel normal. It was good that we had the buffer of a few days before my swim, so they could participate as support crew.

Seasickness can render support crew completely inef-fective. L. Tadeus noted that "when someone goes down with motion sickness, they essentially take another person down with them to tend to them."

This is exactly what happened on a recent night swim across Catalina. The swimmer's wife, the official observer, and the assistant observer were supposed to watch over, feed, and support the swimmer, but they all got seasick and went below to lie down.

The kayaker, who had made about twenty crossings of the Catalina Channel over the past couple of years, was supposed to paddle beside the swimmer. She recognized that conditions were too rough; she didn't think she could control the kayak and was afraid of putting herself and the swimmer at risk. She decided to stay on the boat.

A friend who raced outrigger canoes and had paddled through huge ocean swells offered to be the backup kayaker. This was the first time he had kayaked on a Catalina Channel crossing. He said the waves were breaking all over the place, and it was incredibly rough. He was surprised that the pilot had told the swimmer he could swim. Shortly after he began paddling, a large wave flipped the kayak and tossed him in the water.

The paddler on deck, who had taken on the responsibility of being the person in charge, was focusing intently on the paddler and the swimmer, concerned that she might lose them in the black raging water. The captain recognized that the kayaker needed assistance, left his wheelhouse, and tossed the kayaker a line. The kayaker managed to grab the rope, recover the kayak, flip it back over in the rough seas, climb in, and begin paddling again, but the waves continued to grow.

He tried to communicate with the swimmer to see if he was okay, but the swimmer spoke French and knew only a few words of English. His wife spoke some English and could have translated and checked on him, but she was below deck.

Now the kayaker, who had never gotten seasick, was

feeling like he was going to vomit. He told the kayaker on deck that he was not feeling well. He said that he was bothered by the diesel fumes. She knew it was not unusual for swimmers and crew members to catch whiffs of diesel because of wind shifts and the boat's movement, but the kayaker in the water and swimmer were getting prolonged exposure.

She was beginning to feel seasick, too, but she knew she had to stay on deck to watch the kayaker and the swimmer. She had heard about the swimmer from Switzerland who had disappeared into the waves.

She did not know that breathing fumes accentuated the effects of seasickness. She did not know that something far more critical could be happening—that breathing fumes could cause the swimmer and the kayaker to pass out, aspirate water, and drown. This had happened during a professional swimming race in the 1950s in Argentina. She was not aware that over the years, swimmers had been pulled out of the water after getting sick from the engine fumes.

That's why, in planning a swim and selecting a support boat, the person coordinating the swim should select a boat with a dry stack, which means that the diesel fumes are emitted into the air.

If the kayaker had been able to communicate with the pilot—if she'd had other people on board to watch the swimmer and kayaker—she could have informed the pilot that they were getting fumes, and he could have changed the position of the boat. But at that point, he was doing his best to keep the swimmer on course, using the boat to buffer the waves.

The seas got worse. The swimmer got stung all over his arms by jellyfish and could not communicate that to the kayaker. At four and a half hours into the swim, the swimmer decided that he was done. He climbed out of the water.

This is how L. Tadeus evaluated the swim:

The kayaker on the boat did exactly what she should have done. She conducted some time-critical risk management and realized that the prevailing conditions were beyond her capability level. She knew her go/no-go criteria and opted out. Smart.

The boat support personnel did just the opposite. They probably did not conduct any planning or risk management. If they had, they would have known that weather forecasts for the swim were not promising (risk mitigation).

Additionally, if they were smart (per their physician's guidance), they would have taken prophylactic doses of meclizine starting twelve hours before the swim and every twelve hours throughout the swim to avoid becoming seasick, at a minimum (risk mitigation). They were all mission-ineffective owing to their lack of experience/foresight/knowledge of their limitations. In my humble opinion they put themselves and the swimmer at greater risk.

The swimmer fell somewhere in the middle. He could have done a better job planning, and he could have been less aggressive. He might or might not have known about the weather. He certainly did not know anything about the capabilities of his boat support crew, or he likely would have opted out sooner. It sounds as if he really wanted to swim and pushed a bad position, hoping the weather would improve. At least he finally made a smart call, for everyone's sake.

Clearly, none of them had conducted rehearsals or operations in these meteorological and oceanographic conditions (risk mitigation). The kayaker should have been a better friend to the swimmer and told him no from the start. The swimmer experienced a significant failure to recognize his own limitations. Hopefully, he learned from the experience. Hopefully, *everyone* learned from this experience. Hopefully, they conducted, at a minimum, an informal debrief afterward.

Swimmers and boat crews who are considering taking seasickness medications should consult with their physicians beforehand and let the crew know if they do take them.

Years ago, a group of teenagers and I were attempting to swim across the Catalina Channel. One of our friends who was making the attempt was concerned because she had a history of getting seasick when she rode in small boats in moderate seas. She also had a history of becoming disoriented and hypothermic during training swims.

My father was the physician on board the boat. Without consulting him before the swim, the coach offered us seasickness medication. None of us had ever used these medications before, so we had no way of knowing how they would affect us. Only one swimmer accepted. About halfway across the channel, she became hypothermic and had to be pulled out. I've always wondered if she would have made it across without the medication. All the other swimmers completed the swim.

There will always be new situations on a long swim, things that can't be anticipated. If I were going to consider taking seasickness medications, I would test them out during my workouts, and I would have someone watching over me during those swims. If I had crew members who were susceptible to getting seasick, I would ask them to consult their physicians about the best medication and test it before the swim.

The SEALs are trained to work in extreme seas under challenging conditions. They cannot be ineffective due to motion sickness, or not alert due to meds. They have jobs that have to be done. That's why they "practice like they play." They test seasickness meds during their training, which is crucial to knowing how the meds will affect them.

They understand that seasickness can render support crews completely ineffective. Some seasickness meds cause drowsiness and can affect mental alertness. But for those who get seasick, something is better than nothing. The

SEALs have found that most seasickness meds are like anti-psychotics; the levels have to build up in your system and be continuously maintained. So anybody who thinks he's going to take a pill right before getting on a boat and be fine is wrong. SEALs take them twelve hours in advance, with regular light doses throughout the trip or until they feel comfortable coming down from them. They do it with medical guidance. Medical professionals should always be consulted when someone is considering taking seasickness meds.

Sometimes people are unprepared and get seasick. In one extreme case on a SEAL dive in rough seas, a couple of nurses experienced debilitating seasickness. They came up with an original solution. They administered seasickness meds to each other with rectal suppositories, which provided immediate relief. This method is not for the faint of heart. The SEALs do not recommend transdermal patches at all, because sea spray can wash off or dilute them.

SEALs generally have high tolerances for pain and thus for medications. Seasickness meds, muscle relaxers, and pain meds are for them what daily vitamins are for most other people; Motrin might as well be a sugar pill. Some doctors are medicine averse. But the SEALs operate way out on a pretty far edge of human performance on a routine basis.

TAKING MEDICATIONS DURING A SWIM

Some swimmers take over-the-counter medications during their swims for sore shoulders and aching necks and backs. What many people do not realize is that many of these medications have not been tested on people during strenuous activity. A swim is not the place to experiment.

This information should not be taken as medical advice. Always consult with your physician if you are going to take medications before or during a long swim.

There may be an additional downside to taking medications, according to L. Tadeus:

> If someone is exercising very strenuously, to the point of compromising his biochemistry, then it is possible that even a small dose of medication could push him over the edge to complete compromise and injury.
>
> An anti-inflammatory stops inflammation, and therefore pain, during strenuous activity. The pain is the body's way of saying, "Slow down, you're doing something damaging." The human body was not designed to do all the things we do with it. Overuse injuries are so common for SEALs that we have physical therapy clinics on both coasts. A bigger concern is that anti-inflammatory meds tend to thin the blood, which makes bleeding difficult to stop and has some impact on heat conduction. They can make you bleed out in a traumatic injury scenario or sea-life attack and may lead to hypo- or hyperthermia faster, depending on the dosage. There is also the amplified effect they have on the liver during strenuous activities, especially those that dehydrate you. Fortunately, the liver can regenerate.

I'd never considered that medications could affect the body differently depending upon the person's activity. I spoke with Bob Griffith, one of my support crew, who is a pharmacist. Bob considered it for a moment and said, "Of course your body will be functioning differently when you're strenuously exercising than when you're at rest, and the medications would react differently. What is the best medication you can take for anything?"

"I don't know," I said.

"Nothing, unless you have to," he said.

Chapter 17

Preparation

In everything, preparation is one of the keys to success. Still, there is a growing number of people who want to swim in open water and attempt long swims but do not realize the amount of time and effort it takes to prepare. Recently, a teenager who had climbed the seven summits— the highest mountain on every continent—emailed to ask if I thought he could prepare to swim across the English Channel in a wet suit in six months. He was serious. While I didn't want to dash his enthusiasm, and I realized he was an incredible athlete, I explained that you want to be as prepared as you can to attempt a channel swim, and that it took me years of training with Olympic swimming coaches and another few years to acclimate to the cold. Even in a wet suit, he would lose 80 percent of heat through his head and would cool down in the water. You have to train for open water swimming in the open water, and you have to overprepare, because you never know what challenges you'll encounter during any big swim.

That brings me to the college student from a prestigious university who swam on the women's team and decided to cross the English Channel, probably because her parents had planned a trip to England and Europe and she thought she could fit in the swim. She asked me for advice, but she did not seem at all prepared. She was three months away from her attempt; she had not been training in the open water, had not conditioned to the cold water, and didn't know the name of her pilot.

She swam in rough conditions and made it across in over seventeen hours. She said she blew out both shoulders. Was it worth it? Would she have permanent physical damage?

One reason we condition is to strengthen our bodies and muscles to propel us through the water. We also need that muscle strength to help protect our joints. If we do not work out hard enough or long enough, we can become injured.

If she had taken the swim seriously and conditioned, she might not have blown out her shoulders and might have swum much faster. It comes down to taking the time to be as physically and mentally prepared as you can be.

PHYSICAL TRAINING

When you train in the open water, you need to prepare as much as you can physically before your swim. If you don't, you risk injury, or you might not complete your goal. Open water swimming is very different from pool swimming, where you pretty much know that you'll complete your workout or competitive race. In the open water, there are no guarantees, but your chances of success are a lot higher if you are prepared.

You need to train specifically for the distance you're going to swim. Everyone is different; the amount of time needed to train, the distances needed to swim, and the recovery time between workouts all depends on the individual. It depends on your background and how much you've worked out over the years. It depends on the distance and intensity you've been training, the efficiency of your stroke, and many other factors.

You need to have a coach/trainer and/or a group of swimmers to train with. In some ways, it is similar to the way SEAL trainees train: with instructors who guide, see what they're doing, and help them make corrections if needed.

MENTAL PREPARATION

Once after I gave a lecture to a group of seven hundred prominent people connected with a foundation in Mumbai, India, a ten-year-old boy asked: "When you do the long-distance swims, it takes great physical endurance, but do you think that your ability to achieve the swim is ninety percent mental? That a positive mind-set makes all the difference?"

What a terrific question. My response was that each person finds strength to do a long-distance swim from different sources. For some swimmers, it may be a positive mind-set; for others, it may be that they trained for a long period of time. For me, it is both. If I do not train, I am not prepared mentally, and I do not have confidence in my ability. If being able to achieve a long distance were just about having a positive attitude, I would not train as hard as I do. Positive thoughts and confidence do not physically prepare swimmers for long-distance swims.

For example, you have to be physically and mentally strong to swim the English Channel. Determination is key to completing the swim. You need to have the mind-set that you can complete the swim, especially when the currents are taking you on a tour of the French or English coast or when you are swimming as hard as you can and moving backward. You need to be able to keep going, increase your speed, and continue as long as you have to in order to reach the shore. And do this for hours on end.

For most swimmers, the English Channel is an epic struggle. You never know how the channel is going to challenge you, or what you will find deep within yourself during those challenges.

When you finally get the call and your pilot says, "Your swim's on for tonight," you will experience relief that you're finally getting to go, and you will feel great excitement and uncertainty. What some swimmers do better than others is to push aside these emotions and take a few deep breaths to calm down so they use all their energy for the swim. Some swimmers might have had mentors help them prepare mentally.

Fahmy Attallah was the one who did that for me. He was a friend of a friend, and when we met, when I was fourteen years old, he was a school psychologist in California who, years before, attempted the English Channel five times. Like Yoda, who taught Luke Skywalker how to tap in to the Force and use his instincts to become a warrior, Fahmy was tiny, only five feet tall, and his balding head had white patches of hair above rather large ears. He looked like a grandfather, his brown eyes were bright and his laugh deep and hearty, and he spoke in a clear and calm voice. He was trim, his muscles were well defined, and he was physically strong. He ate a healthy and balanced diet with lots of fruit and vegetables, and he fasted on Sundays to cleanse his system.

When we measured our hands by putting them palm to palm, his were smaller than mine, and his feet were smaller, too. He laughed deeply and told me, "A person's size and age does not matter when you swim across the English Channel. The water is a great equalizer of men and women. You are fourteen years old, but you have been swimming a long time, and you have swum Catalina and you are training with the best Olympic coach, and you are very determined. I know that if you get good weather, you will swim the English Channel and break the men's and women's world records. You have the strength and the determination to do it."

Each time we met for dinner, he asked about my training sessions and how I was doing and whether I was getting enough rest. He asked if I was acclimating to the cold. He worried about the cold, though he tried not to show it. He did not have a chance to condition for the cold water, having grown up in Egypt, and that was a big part of what prevented him from completing his channel swim. He told me I needed to spend a lot of time training for the cold.

Whenever I saw him, he'd say, "The ocean is God's greatest and most beautiful creation." When he did his daily swims off Long Beach, he meditated. He asked what I thought about when I swam, and I told him: I focused on my breath—on the sounds of my inhales and exhales; on the long streams of bubbles released into the water. I felt myself move through the water, and felt how it lifted and flowed around me. For hours I listened to the sounds of my hands capturing water and pulling me across the sea. Sometimes, I felt at one with the water. He told me that I meditated, too.

Fahmy told me detailed stories about training off the shores of Folkestone and in Dover Harbor. His voice would grow dreamy as he said, "The white cliffs are very beautiful. They are so white and high, and you can see them for many, many miles. They are something you never forget."

There was, in all of this, great joy and sadness. He tried not to show his sadness, but sometimes his voice cracked or tightened when he recounted his channel swims and the disappointment he felt when he didn't complete them. He took the discipline and determination from channel swimming and applied them to his life. Those experiences helped him get to England to study at university, and once he graduated, he moved to California to start his practice. He knew that by giving me the gift of his wisdom, he also gave me his dreams to carry on my channel swim.

He told me about the sounds of the waves in Dover Harbor, how the water gently caressed the pebbles. He said the sounds were soothing and they changed with the size of the waves. He described the plaintive calls of the seagulls as they circled high over the white cliffs, the deep moans of the foghorns near the entrance to the harbor, and the blasts of horns of ferryboats and the hovercraft.

Fahmy said that when you enter the water in Dover Harbor, you step down a gentle slope, and you feel the pebbles tumbling over your feet first and then the cold water enveloping you as you walk deeper in. He talked about the way the water felt when he swam, how it was buoyant and how the cold continuously nipped at his skin. He described the course where swimmers trained, and the beach between the ferry and hovercraft terminals, and the pier with a clock tower where swimmers checked their paces and listened to the tower clock chime. He said that this harbor was a special place where swimmers from all over the world met, exchanged knowledge, and often became friends forever.

During one crossing, he swam for twenty-seven hours. He described how tides carried him backward and how he watched the British shore disappear as he drifted toward Belgium. He described the time he got within four hundred yards of the English shore and his crew pulled him out because they thought he was hypothermic.

He set in my mind the attributes that a swimmer needs to swim the English Channel. He said, "You must be a very strong swimmer and have great endurance. You must be able to withstand the cold, waves, and wind for hours on hours. You must be fast to break through currents, and you must be powerful to endure the cold for hours on end." He said he knew I could do this.

Fahmy helped me envision what it would be like. With his memories, he helped fuel my imagination. At night before I went to sleep, I heard the sounds of the waves in Dover Harbor and the calls of the seagulls. The English

Channel has not changed much in all these years. Neither have the coasts of England and France.

It always helps to find other swimmers who have swum the English Channel, who will sit down and give you their time and share their experiences and help you mentally prepare for your swim.

What most swimmers not do know is that there can be an emotional letdown after a big swim. Mark, a swimmer who'd completed the Catalina Channel an hour or so before our meeting, said he felt a sense of accomplishment but also, "Completing the swim was bittersweet. I felt somewhat sad," he said.

Most swimmers go through a period of elation, and then they have a difficult time unwinding and sometimes sleeping after a big swim. It usually takes some time for the achievement to sink in, and a few days or weeks before swimmers feel a letdown.

After I swam the English Channel at age fifteen and broke the men's and women's records, I was at a loss. I didn't have any idea what I wanted to do next. Fortunately, Davis Hart, a great swimmer and coach from Springfield, Massachusetts, swam across the English Channel a couple of months after I did. He broke my record and gave me a new focus. I decided to train hard and return to the channel to try to break his time. When I achieved that goal the following summer, I already had an idea of what I wanted to do next. I could use the momentum from each success to work on larger goals.

It is important to have a plan for what you will do if you succeed at your goal and what to if you don't.

Chapter 18

Going In and Out of Consciousness

Chloë McCardel, an Australian swimmer who completed an amazing double crossing of the English Channel, decided to return to England to attempt a triple crossing. She was a fast and powerful swimmer with magnificent endurance, and she had the very best crew. Paul, her husband, was part of her support crew and had a strong open water swimming background. Murph Renford was on her swim as well. He had swum across the English Channel himself, and as a boy, he had accompanied Des Renford, his father, on his English Channel swim. Over the years, Murph had mentored other Australian swimmers. Chloë also selected Reg and Ray Brickell for her triple crossing attempt. They were two of the most experienced English Channel pilots.

As boys, Reg and Ray worked with their father, Reg Sr., on their fishing boat and during English Channel attempts. They learned about the sea and about the swimmers, and they all took great pride in Reg Sr.'s achievement of guiding the most world record–breaking swimmers.

Reg and Ray had been on Des's solo swims and attempts for a double. They had learned from the best, and they upgraded their technology whenever they could to give their swimmer an additional edge. Reg Jr. had been on my English Channel swim, as well as David Yudovin's successful swim. Even though Chloë had the best support team, something went wrong.

Over breakfast months later, Murph told me about Chloe's swim. He was concerned about what had happened. It really bothered him that neither he nor Paul had recognized that Chloë was in trouble. He wanted to talk about it and make other swimmers and crew more aware and their swims safer.

Murph said that Chloë completed the first lap of her English Channel triple in just over nine hours and three minutes, the fastest crossing of the season. When she reached shore, she looked happy, strong, and very capable. The crew watched her push off the French shore and swim back toward England. Paul watched her along with Murph on deck. Reg and Ray had a camera fixed on Chloë at all times and watched her from the pilot's cabin. Chloë and Paul agreed with the current status quo, whereby the pilot has the final decision of when to pull a swimmer out—not the observer or support crew.

The sea conditions were good. Chloë swam in 60-degree F (15.5-degree C) water. She stopped to tread water and eat or drink roughly every twenty to thirty minutes. Reg met with Paul to discuss her progress and condition, and the observers listened to the conversation nearly every time. Paul and Chloë had tested an internal core temperature machine in the weeks leading into the channel attempt, but unfortunately, they had to abandon the device days before the swim due to technical difficulties.

Around the twelve-hour mark, Paul noticed that Chloë was getting cranky during her feed stops. Murph hoped that she was just fatigued and would swim through it and be better on the other side. He was so seasick that he went below to sleep. When he came back on deck an hour later, Paul said that Chloë was not swimming her best but was still making good progress; her stroke rate had slowed only slightly. However, Reg and Ray noted that Chloë was making much slower progress on the slack tide. They knew she was capable of swimming faster. Her stoke rate had dropped to the low sixties, compared with her normal sixty-six strokes per minute. She was unaware of her stroke rate during the swim.

Her budget allowed for only two support crew and two observers for a marathon swim that could have lasted up to forty hours. At times Murph became very seasick and had to relinquish his duties to Paul. The observers were a father and daughter. They were there to monitor Chloë's progress and to advise the pilot and crew if she were in danger and needed to be pulled out of the water. Murph said that the father seemed competent but the daughter really had no idea of her job. In fact, at times she was on the other side of the boat, out of Chloë's view, while her father was below sleeping.

Murph said that he got very worried when "Chloe had a really big vomit at one particular feed stop." He thought that was what began her downward spiral. It had happened to him on his first attempt across the Catalina Channel. He had eaten a pasta dish and thought he might have food poisoning, but he started off anyway and began vomiting on the swim and continued to be sick and ultimately had to get out of the water. Murph said, "As the swim progressed further, she had difficulties consuming all one hundred percent of her feeds." Chloë disagreed. She said that her swim was different from Murph's; the one feed when she was sick, despite losing approximately ten minutes in speed, had a minimal effect on the rest of her swim and did not contribute to her drop in core temperature down the track. In fact, her stroke rate decreased rapidly after a cold front set in on the channel, which was many hours after she had vomited. Paul and Chloë believe she was consuming 90 percent of her feeds, which is standard for her marathon swimming. Paul puts about 110 percent of what she should consume into each feed, to be conservative. The experts Chloë and Paul spoke to believe the cold front was the cause of her severe hypothermia.

Murph and Paul, channel swimmers themselves, and the observers who were experts, did not recognize that she was in trouble. Chloë did not show any outward signs of hypothermia. She wasn't shivering or slurring her speech. They knew her pace was slower, but they just thought she was going through a bad spot, as often happens on channel swims when the swimmer gets tired or struggles against a current. Murph believed that because of her two previous English Channel swims—forty-seven hours in total—she could pull off the triple. And with her track record, who could blame him?

The perplexing thing for Murph was that Chloë never complained; she was prepared to keep swimming. Murph said, "Reg also noted that Chloë was still six miles (9.6 kilometers) off completing the double. This meant a possible six hours for her to get to England, and the way she was swimming, it just wasn't on. Paul, with all on board, agreed that the swim was over. Chloë was the only one not on the same page, partly because of the condition she was in and partly because she is just so bloody tough. She was only swimming sixteen hundred meters an hour on a slack tide when she averages four thousand meters an hour, and from a stroke rate that dropped from sixty-six to fifty-two strokes a minute over the last ninety minutes, it was clear that the triple was not on and that a double was not even an option."

Murph and Paul called her over to the swim ladder located at the stern of the boat. Chloë swam over and looked at the ladder but wouldn't touch it. She knew as soon as she touched it, the swim was over. This is the most difficult part for a swimmer, when she wants to continue but can't. It is equally hard on the crew. But Murph and Paul realized that Chloë had reached her limit.

Finally, Murph convinced Chloë, she grabbed the ladder, and the crew pulled her out of the water and onto the deck. They immediately wrapped her in blankets, and she seemed okay. She fell asleep with her head resting on Paul's shoulder, and when they reached the Folkestone harbor, she woke up, but she was not mentally coherent and could not walk without a lot of support. Paul and Murph realized that Chloë was in very bad shape.

Murph realized it would take too long for an ambulance to respond. He and Paul put Chloë in a car and raced to the hospital. A critical-care physician attended to her. He said that she had been going in and out of consciousness and aspirating water throughout her swim. The water she aspirated had gone into her lungs. She spent two days in intensive care before she was well enough to be released from the hospital. The doctor told them that if Chloë had been in the water another half an hour, she could have died. What concerned Murph and the other team members was that Chloë was so programmed to complete the swim, she would have continued without realizing the danger she was in.

Murph's concerns became mine. Like Murph, I wanted to know if there were better ways of monitoring a swimmer. Because of Reg's experience, he recognized that Chloë was getting into trouble long before everyone else did, but he wanted to give her the benefit of the doubt.

L. Tadeus often works with colleagues and trainees who are pushing themselves to their limits, and because the SEAL instructors have to know where those limits are, I asked him what he thought might have happened during Chloë's swim.

He said he thought that the swimmer might have been asleep while swimming. It had happened to him during Hell Week, a time when SEAL trainees go through extreme mental and physical training and stress, with limited sleep.

He was conducting an event called "the base tour." Essentially, the trainees ran around Naval Amphibious

Base Coronado for three hours. He remembered only bits and pieces of it, because he was running while he was sleeping. He explained that the mind does what it perceives it needs to do on all levels. If you need to keep swimming, the mind will allow that, as long as it can accomplish other critical functions simultaneously.

He said that a competent doctor would have known to ask questions that required reasoning. Even if Chloë had a very sharp mind, eventually, she would lose the ability to problem-solve and reason. He gave the following recommendations:

~ Don't ask the swimmer what year it is. Ask what year last year was or what year was two years ago.
~ Don't ask the swimmer what day of the week it is. Ask what day two days ago was. Make her think. Make her say a riddle.

He continued:

There are tons of neurological deficits that occur in these situations. Here's an example: When our trainees surface after a free swimmer ascent, we require them to say specifically, "I feel fine!" Not "I feel good," "I'm cool," "Awesome," or anything else. If a diver is suffering from arterial gas embolism, it will manifest itself in an inability to pronounce two consecutive words beginning with the letter F. It would not surprise me if there were a hypothermia-related analogue to this.

Chloë's speed drop was a pretty good indicator in and of itself. Anyone watching closely enough would have seen her aspirating water routinely—another big indicator. Despite the crew's experience, they were on quite a long journey; their rotation plan to keep topside safety observers fresh and alert was not adequate.

If a swim is long, the swimmer will need sleep at some point. It baffles me how someone can fall asleep while running or swimming. The SEALs believe that the mind separates things into layers. There are things that the mind controls without conscious thought (breathing, sleeping, sweating, pumping blood), and there are things that require conscious thought. Conscious decisions can blur the line between these barriers.

Researchers have discovered that we can decide what we do even when the brain is telling us we should do something else. A father can grab a burning pot and throw it in the sink because he knows it will save his family from death—in spite of the fact that his brain is telling him not to touch it. A swimmer will consciously complete a channel swim in spite of severe shoulder pain indicating that overuse injury is occurring.

So the SEALS regularly have their trainees continue to train past certain points; they aren't ordered to do it. They just train to the point of unconsciousness, when what their brain is telling them to do is get to the surface and breathe. Human limits are very far from where we perceive them to be. Many times it boils down to desire.

The key for us is that the SEALS are the elite maritime force. They have incredible training, knowledge, and standards, and their instructors and leadership create safety nets that enable trainees and SEALs to push themselves as far as they can go, so that they are extremely prepared for their missions. In open water swimming, swimmers push themselves to their limits. The support crew for the a swim has to know how far a swimmer can go, when the swimmer is in trouble, or when the swimmer has reached his limits. There's always a balance, but it is often elusive to know where that is. That's why swimmers need to know their own capabilities and have support crew who know their histories. Swimmers may not realize when they have reached their limit, and this decision may have to be made for them without their help. Swimmers cannot remain objective.

DEEP MIND "THING"

There is a point on some swims when I've been so deep in my mind that I am not aware of what's going on around me. I know that other open water swimmers have had a similar experience. It's different from daydreaming, when your mind floats from one topic to another. When you are engaged in the deep mind "thing," you are going much deeper into your thoughts.

SEALs experience the deep mind thing. Some do it when they swim or run and emerge from it and wonder where the last couple of miles went. The SEALs call this "going to your happy place."

They discovered that the deep mind thing sometimes happens at even a slightly deeper level for trainees during Hell Week. It's as if they are experiencing two different realities simultaneously, and when they emerge from deep mind into reality, they aren't quite sure which is real for a while.

This disconnection—perhaps learned through intense training—carries over for some people to everyday life. Are there times when you've been driving and can remember only the beginning and the destination but not the drive itself? Have you ever emerged from deep mind to find yourself in a situation that only a quick reaction would get you out of? Ever find yourself too close to oncoming traffic and have to jerk the wheel to navigate back to your lane? What are the potential consequences on a swim?

The SEALs have learned that there is something all swimmers can do that doesn't interfere with rhythm. It requires neurological fitness; and it gives a positive indication to surface support. Also, it can't become muscle memory, so that a swimmer does it even when practically or actually unconscious.

The SEALs use a periodic interaction, visual or physical, that forces the trainee/swimmer to problem-solve in order to come up with the correct signals. They recognize that it's difficult to do it in a way that doesn't interrupt the swimmer's rhythm, so they create a meaningful interaction between the swimmer and the surface so that support can truly assess the swimmer's physical and mental state. That might come in the form of a thirty-second break every ten minutes during which the swimmer has to answer questions that require thought. For example, what was last year's date? What was yesterday's date? What is tomorrow's date? What is the date before your birthday? Who was the last president? The questions require consciousness, brief thought, and problem solving, but aren't as complicated as a Rubik's Cube. The trainees respond with very brief answers.

The SEALs routinely use hand signals to convey information. One instructor suggested that swimmers work with their crews to develop hand signals to provide answers to questions. The questions could be asked over a diver recall transducer, or underwater speaker, so the swimmer can hear the questions underwater. The answers can be given while taking a stroke. There are a lot of signals that are possible with the hands and fingers.

SLEEP

There are open water swimmers who attempt swims that last for over twenty-four hours, and there are triathletes who attempt double Ironmans that take over twenty hours to complete. If swimmers are using the Channel Swimming Association rules, they aren't allowed to climb into the support boat or have any kind of artificial assistance during their swims, and they are not able to stop and sleep.

No doubt, these huge swims and triathlons test minds and bodies, but it's worth taking a look at how the SEALs train, to understand what sleep deprivation does to the mind and body, and why it's so important to integrate sleep into the training cycle.

The instructors know that there is a specific amount of sleep that trainees must get. This was not always the case. For earlier SEAL trainee classes, sleep was incidental. One SEAL remembered that during Hell Week, the trainees got forty-five minutes of sleep one night—but not because they needed sleep. The instructors put the trainees down to rewarm them, because the air temperature had dropped to 37 degrees F (2.7 degrees C). Now very brief sleep periods are programmed into the schedule, based on scientific research.

These days instructors take things much slower and conduct a lot more medical monitoring. They have observed that sleep deprivation makes trainees much more susceptible to hypothermia, hyperthermia, hypoglycemia, viral gastroenteritis, and swimmer-induced pulmonary edema. Sleep deprivation also increases the risk of injury, despite a healthy diet. Instructors have found that the body needs time to shut down and conduct maintenance. Sleep deprivation compromises an immune system.

Five days of straight sleep deprivation is about as long as an instructor would take someone before letting him shut down for a bit. After that, they start risking psychotic episodes. Hallucinations usually start between the third and fourth days. Getting enough sleep before any open water swim will increase your chances of success.

Chapter 19

Motivations

While the example below concerns advanced open water swimming, the information about motivations and goals applies to all open water swimmers.

Dave, my brother, coached David Yudovin; Dan Slosberg; another swimmer; and me. He launched our open water swimming lives.

Dan Slosberg completed a single Catalina Channel crossing and became the first person to swim a double. David Yudovin swam across the English Channel; became the first person to swim across the Tsugaru Channel between Honshu and Hokkaido, Japan; and became the first to swim between the islands of Indonesia and between some of the Hawaiian Islands.

The other swimmer in our group was faster than any of us. He was incredibly talented and churned out miles in rough waters without getting tired. When he decided to swim across the Catalina Channel, he was in top shape, or so we all thought. He pushed offshore and swam strongly for about ten strokes before stopping abruptly.

Dave asked if he was cold, sick, injured, or scared. The

swimmer said that he was okay, he just didn't want to do the swim. Without any hesitation, he climbed out of the water.

Dave later tried to talk to him about it, but he never wanted to talk. He said only that he felt he let us down and let himself down.

We tried to figure out what happened and came to the conclusion that he psyched himself out. He was physically ready, but something wasn't there mentally. He left the salt water for over thirty years but reappeared to compete in some long races. We still talk about him and wonder why he didn't try again. Maybe it was as simple as he just didn't want to do it.

From all the years of watching open water swimmers, being on other people's swims, coaching, or advising from a distance, I've learned that whether it's your first swim or the fiftieth, whether it's a short or long swim, the swim needs to be your goal, not someone else's. You can't do these swims to make someone else proud.

You have to swim because you want to swim, and you have to want to accomplish it more than anything else. You also have to stay away from negative influences—people who do not support your goals—and you need to have trust in your coach and his or her ability to support your goal.

The mind plays an enormous role in the outcome of a swim.

SUCCESS

There's nothing like training, preparing, researching, finding the best crew, working with local people and learning from them, waiting for the tides and weather, finally getting the chance to swim, and succeeding. It is thrilling. You achieved your biggest goal. All the effort was worthwhile, and it is so satisfying. The success boosts your confidence, and after a week or two to recover, you begin to think about what you will do next. What few people talk about is the letdown, even if you have succeeded.

Last year, Brad McVetta, a triathlete who became an open water swimmer, completed the Catalina Channel crossing. His and his crew met with me for lunch at a Mexican restaurant. His smile was so big, his eyes were bright, and he was very happy with his success. His overall feeling was that he'd met his goal, but he seemed reflective while ordering his food and waiting for it to arrive.

I asked, "How are you doing?"

He smiled and said, "The swim was the most difficult athletic event I've ever done. It doesn't even compare to a triathlon." He was tired and sore, but not as sore as he'd expected, and he said he felt a little sad that the swim was over.

I said, "That's usual. You put so much effort into what you were doing, and then it's over. That big goal that was right before you for so long is now behind you."

Brad agreed and said, "You build up such a sense and vision of what it will be like when you land, during training, that it can't possibly be that way when you do. And also during the swim, you are wrestling with thoughts of will you make it, and then at some point your will just finally silences those negatives. And shortly after, your mind arrives onshore, but you may be miles away. I never intentionally looked up to see how close I was. My celebration started then, and I swam for another thirty minutes, and by the time I landed, I was partied out."

I asked if he had other plans looming on the horizon, and he said he was thinking about other swims and other goals. I told him that was very wise. Many swimmers get so caught up in achieving one big goal that they don't have any idea what they will do next, and they are lost for a while.

Brad needed to take a nice long hot shower and relax and savor all the things that he enjoyed during the swim. I suggested that he write about it as soon as he could, so that he wouldn't lose the experience.

A few months later, I checked on him. He sounded even happier and more satisfied with his Catalina accomplishment. He was working toward new goals in swimming and in life.

SUCCESS IN UNSUCCESSFUL SWIMS

Sometimes the goal is further than you can reach.

When swims don't work out, for whatever reason, it is normal to be disappointed or even depressed. Sometimes it's hard to figure out what didn't work and then decide whether to try again or do something else. It is very disappointing and hard to deal with not completing something that you've worked so hard on. It's important to take time to process what happened.

During training for my first English Channel swim, I met Sandra Blewett in Dover Harbor. Sandy was from New Zealand and had attempted the English Channel the year before. She got within seven miles (11.2 kilometers) of the French coast, where the current can be problematic, and she couldn't make it in.

She was about six years older than I was. It was nice to have someone around my age in the water. Most of the other swimmers were much older—in their twenties, thirties, and forties. We talked about our training and our plans for the swim.

Sandy was determined and focused, but once again, she didn't complete the swim. Once again, she got within seven miles (11.2 kilometers) of the French coast and couldn't finish. I felt really bad for her.

We still stay in touch, and recently, she asked if I would coach her to swim across the Catalina Channel.

She worked very hard and did whatever I asked of her, but she was freaked out by seaweed. I knew that she had to get over it. When you swim across the Catalina Channel, you usually run into seaweed at the start and the finish. I told her that if she was afraid, it would take energy away from her forward movement.

We swam half-mile (0.8-kilometer) laps together off Santa Barbara, parallel to the beach, near large kelp beds. Sandy was not pleased with the arrangement, but I explained that we needed to do it so she would get used to it.

After a few laps, she began to relax, and then I coaxed her over to the kelp and showed her how to reverse her stroke if she got tangled in it, how to grab hold of it to pull herself forward, and how to float on top of it. We continued swimming, and she got caught in kelp and jumped. She wanted to get out but knew that if she did, I wouldn't coach her for Catalina. She was annoyed at me, but she continued swimming, and she got through the kelp. And then we dove under it and made sure to clear it before we surfaced.

Sandy had it in her. She continued her training and completed the Catalina Channel in something like fifteen hours. She was pleased with her success and confident that she could complete the English Channel. She asked me to coach her. We met in England and waited a couple of weeks for good weather and tides. On the day of her attempt, the seas were calm and she was ready, but when she got within seven miles of shore, she suddenly looked disoriented and her stroke rate dropped to zero. We had to pull her out of the water.

We discussed her swim for a couple of days and couldn't figure out what had gone wrong. It seemed to be something about getting within the seven-mile (11.2 kilometer) distance. Her times had varied on the other attempts by two to three hours. She physically had gone farther on the Catalina Channel. I suggested that she try training in colder water, doing longer swims, using different foods, and interval training to sustain a faster speed and get across the channel faster.

She was very disappointed, and I felt bad that she hadn't made it. It seemed like it was something physiological, though I wasn't an expert.

Before she attempted another crossing, I told her, she had to figure out what she needed to change. I suggested talking to other channel swimmers who could offer more insights.

A few days later, I left to swim across Lake Geneva and heard two weeks later that Sandy had attempted the channel again, gotten within seven miles (11.2 kilometers), and had to be pulled out.

After that, Sandy stayed in England for years. She worked as a swimming coach and then on board a ferry boat that crossed the English Channel two to three times a day. Something like twenty years later, she completed the English Channel swim. It was her life's achievement.

Mind-set plays an enormous role in whether you succeed. Trainees experience a big letdown if they don't complete their SEAL training. L. Tadeus recounted his experience while working with the trainees:

> We see it all the time with trainees who do not complete Hell Week. It really boils down to mental resiliency. Somewhere in everyone's mind there is this very fine line—the normal. On one side of the line, a setback motivates them to try harder—the "if knocked down, I will get back up every time" mentality. On the opposite side of the line, a setback demotivates them. The severity of the setback determines how far away from the normal line they are pushed. In extreme cases, the person can find disaster on both sides of the line. A person in the first category may keep getting up when he should probably stay down.

We have noticed a recent trend of trainees concealing life-altering injuries just to stay in the program. A person in the other category may never try again or become so despondent that he becomes suicidal.

We see the whole spectrum here.

Chapter 20

The English Channel Charts, Contacts, and Pilots

The English Channel, also known as the Strait of Dover, in a straight line is a twenty-one-mile channel between Shakespeare Beach, England, and Cape Gris Nez, France. The English Channel stopped the Spanish Armada and Hitler from invading Britain. For many, the English Channel is the Mount Everest of long-distance swimming, though there are more people who have climbed Mount Everest than have swum the English Channel. Roughly 150 to 300 swimmers will attempt the English Channel each year. In a good year, about 20 percent of the solo swimmers and 60 percent of the relay swimmers reach the other shore. The success of channel swims, like Everest climbs, is tied to nature. The outcome of a swim depends upon the tide, sea, and weather.

An English Channel swim is planned around the phases of the moon and the weather. During the month, there are two tides that occur: the spring tide and the neap tide. The spring tide is when the difference between high and low water is the greatest. It happens when the moon is either new or full, and the sun, moon, earth are all in alignment. When this occurs, the gravitational pull on the earth's oceans is strengthened, which causes the greatest rise and fall in the tidal level. The spring tide causes the water to move more and the current to be considerably stronger.

The neap tide occurs at the first and last quarter of the moon, when the tide generating of the sun and moon are opposite each other. This produces the smallest rise and fall in the tides. The neap tides occur twice a month, when the sun and moon are at right angles to the earth. The gravitational pull on the earth's oceans is weakened because the sun and moon come from two different directions. During the neap tide, you have less water movement and weaker current. A solo swimmer will attempt an English Channel swim on a neap tide. A relay team comprised of two to six swimmers may make an attempt on the start of the spring tide or the end of the spring tide.

TIDAL CHARTS

Spring tides and neap tides alternate, so that you will have two spring tides and two neap tides in a month. One week the spring tide occurs; the next week, the neap tide; the following week, the spring tide; and the last week of the month, the neap tide. This tidal sequence is important because there are only two weeks during the month when solo swimmers should attempt English Channel swims.

When you look at a tidal chart, the difference between high and low water tells you how fast the tidal current is moving. If there is a great numerical difference between high and low water, you will know that time period has the strongest water movement between high and low water. You want to select a tide when there is the least difference between high and low water.

For the English Channel, most swimmers begin their swim an hour before slack water or just at slack. Slack water is the end of a tide, when the current is tailing off and about to change to the opposite direction. The tidal change does not happen all at once; it builds gradually, until it reaches full strength in the middle of the tide, and then tapers off.

Before GPS, when swimmers swam the English Channel, their courses resembled an inverted S, and this reflected the tidal movement. The direct distance between England and France is twenty-one miles, but the first time I swam the English Channel, I swam thirty miles; the second time, I swam thirty-three. These were typical distances for the English Channel back then, but if you look at a swimmer's chart from a recent swim, the distance will most likely be twenty-one to twenty-two miles. This accuracy has enabled swimmers to complete their swims in much faster times.

YOU WANT TO SWIM THE ENGLISH CHANNEL?

Swimming across channels is far more complex than swimming alongshore. Nature's forces play larger roles in water movement in the ocean. Currents, tides, temperatures, salinity, the earth's rotation, and moving weather systems all have a great impact. Landmasses pinch, deflect, accelerate, funnel, and buffer the water's path. Below the water's surface, undersea mountains, rifts, reefs, canyons, and sandbars, the irregular crucible of sandy beaches or rocky shores, all alter the water's motion.

You swim through hues of liquid gold and blue toward a distant horizon where dreams and destiny meet. You feel the power of your arms and legs and the winds and waves as they flow and rush everywhere around you. You swim through darkness into light, cross shifting seas and calm ones. You focus on the gains you make and overcome the losses. You dig deep into the sea, and into your mind, resolving to overcome the waves, tides, and any barrier. With skill and guidance from your crew, you reach beyond yourself. It is not a simple swim. It's not achieved alone or in haste. It's done with conscious acts of kindness and inspiration. And at the end, the celebration is shared with everyone. It is with their skill and guidance that you have traveled beyond your reach, and together you have spanned a great distance, shared hopes and dreams, and crossed from one great landmass to another.

HOW DO YOU MAKE CONTACT?

Some of the questions that you will want to consider are: Is it important for you to have your swim verified? Do you want or need to use an established organization?

Most swimmers who swim across the English Channel become members of the Channel Swimming Association (CSA) or the Channel Swimming and Piloting Federation (CSPF). Both groups were established to authenticate, observe, and verify English Channel swims. The CSA is the more traditional association. Their rules require that a swimmer begin from shore and completely clear the water to finish. Swimmers are permitted to wear only a swimsuit, a swim cap, goggles, and some type of grease. The CSPF was established to cater to the more unorthodox crossings, like rowing or canoeing, and they assist swimmers wearing wet suits.

Both associations have a list of pilots to escort the swimmer for a channel crossing. There are six active pilots in the CSA and nine active pilots in the CSPF. Swimmers are required to have a pilot for their English Channel swim and need to become a member of the Channel Swimming Association or the Channel Swimming and Piloting Federation if they want to attempt the swim and have it authenticated.

There are fees associated with becoming a member. Because the fees change annually, it is best to check the websites: www.channelswimmingassociation.com and www.channelswimming.net. The websites provide listings of and contact information for pilots. Pilots are essential for English Channel swims and are registered with the British Coast Guard. For safety reasons, the British Coast Guard limits the number of boats that can assist swimmers to twelve a day.

Pilots charge fees to guide swimmers across the English Channel. The fees vary. Pilots also charge according to the length of a swim—for instance, if you are swimming a single crossing, a double crossing, or a relay attempt. They require a deposit, a booking fee, and the remainder of the payment before or after the swim, depending upon the pilot.

Many of the English Channel pilots are fishermen. Some learned how to fish from their father and grandfather, and they know the English Channel like a friend and an old foe. The English Channel pilots are like the Sherpas who guide climbers up Mount Everest. The same way Sherpas know the mountains and weather, the pilots read the tides, currents, weather patterns, and local conditions. Pilots help swimmers determine the best day to swim. It is essential to find the best pilot possible: the one who is the most experienced, qualified, and compatible with the swimmer.

As in everything, some pilots are better than others. A miscalculation on the part of a pilot can make the difference between completing and not completing the swim. It is important to select a pilot who has taken swimmers successfully across the English Channel.

SELECTING A PILOT

Because of the enormous interest in swimming across the English Channel, there are more swimmers than support boats. Swimmers who decide they want to attempt the swim need to book with a pilot two to three years in advance. The best way to find a pilot is to ask swimmers who have completed the English Channel about their experiences and whom they recommend. Most pilots will book four to five solo swimmers and one relay team on one tide. Some pilots will also double-book swimmers, promising the tides to two swimmers on one day, hoping to get one swimmer across and then return to England to escort a second swimmer in the same twenty-four-hour period. This is not the best arrangement for either swimmer.

Weather plays a critical role in a swimmer's opportunity to attempt a swim. If you have booked the tide and are in the number one position, you have the first chance of attempting the swim on the first day of the tide. If the weather is not good on the first day, you are still number one on the tide; you have the option to attempt the swim on the second tide; and if you can't swim because of weather, you have the option to swim on the third tide. If the weather still is not good, you have the option for the fourth tide, and ultimately, the fifth day. If the weather causes a no-swim, the swimmer can choose to go on the next set of available tides, or when the pilot has availability. The swimmer discusses these options with the pilot. The pilot fees are not refunded but are carried over to the following year. Each pilot is in charge of his own bookings, and it is worth asking before the swim what will happen if the weather causes a no-swim.

One of the problems with being in number two, three, four, or five position on the tide is that you have less of a chance to attempt a swim; however, a fair number of swimmers cancel their swims for one reason or another, and that may open up a spot.

You need to determine which pilot will work the best with you. The pilot must care about the swimmer. Most pilots take great pride in assisting swimmers and do everything they can to help a swimmer succeed.

When I swam the English Channel, Reg Brickell Sr. was my pilot, and his son Reg was his assistant. I was not as informed then as I am now. The Channel Swimming Association gave me a list of pilots, and I went down the list until I found someone who answered the phone.

By great fortune, it was Reg Brickell. Reg had taken the most record-breaking swimmers across the English Channel, and even though I was only fifteen years old, he took me seriously and understood that my goal was to break the world records for men and women. He did everything he could to help me realize that goal.

Reg watched over me intently for the entire swim, his fair brow often wrinkled with concern, his blue eyes alternating between our course and me swimming beside the pilothouse. He leaned over and checked on me countless times and often smiled and gave me a thumbs-up that I was right on pace. Toward the end of my first channel crossing, when we hit currents so strong that we were being pushed backward, Reg told me I needed to swim faster, and for the last hour, he cheered me on. He drew upon all of his experience and kept working to find solutions to get me through the currents. He made all the difference and enabled me to break the men's and women's world records twice. His sons, Reg and Ray, have followed in his footsteps and are among the top echelon of channel swimming pilots.

There are great pilots who care a great deal about swimmers and the outcome of the swim, and there are pilots who are motivated by the business of the swim. Steve Riches, who grew up in England and now lives in California, decided to do a relay swim across the English Channel with a group of friends. All of them were good swimmers. Based on a recommendation from another swimmer friend, they booked with a pilot. They told him that they were not interested in breaking the record for the relay. They just wanted to complete the swim.

During the relay crossing, Steve said that he stopped in

the channel to look around and take in the full experience. He joked with his friends who were watching him from the boat, and they laughed together.

The pilot shouted at Steve to get moving, and when Steve didn't, he began cursing at him. The pilot said he was wasting petrol and the pilot's time. Steve said they had paid in full for the boat and pilot's service, and they would take as much time as they needed to do the swim and enjoy it. They did just that.

Looking back, Steve said, "It's so important to have a good pilot, as it's a once-in-a-lifetime experience for most people." If he were to swim the channel again, he said, he would spend more time finding a pilot who was compatible with his goals.

The English Channel pilots provide their service as a safety net for the swimmer. They protect swimmers from shipping and fog, and guide them, and are there for support. If swimmers are in trouble during a swim, the pilot makes the decision about whether to let them continue swimming or to pull them out of the water.

Some swimmers have their crew video them to enable them so later they can examine what they could do to improve on future channel crossings. They have found this to be a very effective tool.

Chapter 21

Catalina and Other Channel Swims

THE CATALINA CHANNEL SWIM

The Catalina Channel Swimming Federation in California was established to observe swims across the Catalina Channel, also known as the San Pedro Channel. The federation observes and verifies Catalina Channel swims. The group cares about the swimmers and does a lot to support swimmers and the growth of the sport.

At this point, Catalina Channel Swimming Federation (see Sources for website address; page 301) works with two different pilots who own two different boats. The two pilots are hired by the swimmers.

The setup for hiring escort boats for the Catalina Channel is very different from that of the English Channel. With the Catalina Channel, a swimmer is given one day to attempt the swim. Murph Renford attempted a Catalina Channel crossing recently. He said that with the English Channel, "you are given a window of opportunity. You get to swim on a tide, depending on your position on the tide. And if you can't get off before the neaps end, you have the option of going on a spring tide or returning the following year to attempt the swim." With the English Channel swim, the pilot decides whether or not you will swim. With the Catalina Channel swim, the swimmer has to decide whether or not to swim, and you only get one day. If you don't go on that day, you get your money refunded and can come back the following year.

> There is so much pressure, especially when you come all the way from Australia. There's a lot of expense in travel, hotels, food, and the crew. My pilot told me that my swim would be in the most marginal conditions he had ever taken anyone across, and I had to decide whether to go. I decided to go, and the waves were breaking all over the place. They couldn't find a direction, and I couldn't get a rhythm. I would get slapped in the head by one wave and in the face by another. Tony, my friend, was having a hard time just staying on his paddleboard. We had a backup boat, and it was getting so thrashed that the captain decided to return to the harbor.
>
> After the first hour, I wondered what would be an acceptable time for a failure. I really didn't think I could keep going. But I did. I'm not that mentally tough, but I kept going. I told Tony, "Let's smash ourselves for an hour," meaning let's sprint. Tony couldn't believe it, and he said, "Murph, slow down," but I sprinted anyway.

Murph completed the swim in nine hours and thirteen minutes. He was very satisfied with his success, but he would be the first to say that having only one day to attempt a swim puts the swimmer in a bad position. He said, "You take risks you would not normally take."

The boat support guides the swimmer and, along with the crew, makes sure the swimmer is safe. If a swimmer is being pressured to swim in far less than ideal conditions, that is not a good situation.

In the last couple of years, there have been record numbers of people planning the swim. This year there were more than fifty, and with the limited number of tides and days of fair weather, it would be good for the sport if there were more pilots available.

One friend decided to swim across the Catalina Channel with a relay. They didn't book a pilot with the federation because they didn't want to pay the fees; instead, they asked a capable friend to be their pilot. They swam under the English Channel swimming rules, started the swim on a great day, and completed it. Their swim was not verified by the Catalina Channel Swimming Association, but that did not matter to them. They went through all the proper procedures and knew what they had achieved. They were satisfied with their success.

THE SANTA BARBARA CHANNEL SWIM

The Santa Barbara Channel, north of the Catalina Channel, is becoming another popular place for open water swims. Scott Zornig, the president of the Santa Barbara Swimming Association and a very successful open water swimmer who has swum between many of the islands in the Santa Barbara Channel, has been encouraging open water swimmers to swim there. Scott has labeled them "the Southern California Eight," consisting of swims from each of the Channel Islands: Anacapa (12.4 miles; 19.9 kilometers), Santa Cruz (19.0 miles; 30.5 kilometers), Catalina (20.4 miles; 32.8 kilometers), San Miguel (25.9 miles; 41.6 kilometers), Santa Rosa (27.5 miles; 44.2 kilometers), Santa Barbara (37.7 miles; 60.6 kilometers), San Clemente (54.4 miles; 87.5 kilometers), and San Nicolas Island (61.2 to 69.3 miles, or 98.4 to 111.5 kilometers, depending on course). For more information about the association and the swims, take a look at www.santabarbarachannelswim.org.

FINDING PILOTS FOR
THE CATALINA CHANNEL AND OTHER SWIMS

In 1972, Dave, my older brother, decided to swim across the Catalina Channel. Dave was a nationally ranked swimmer and had trained with Don Gambril, who had been the U.S. Olympic swim coach. In the 1970s there weren't any pilots taking swimmers across the Catalina Channel, but John Sonnichsen, who had been involved in open water swimming since the 1950s, offered to help.

John had coached swimmers and had supported some professional swimmers during the 1950s. He understood swimmers, as well as the tides and currents. He knew how to read the water, and he could tell when swimmers were making progress and when they were struggling.

John offered to help Dave find a competent pilot for his swim and to accompany them on the swim and work with the pilot. John found Mickey Pitman, in San Pedro, California. Mickey was a professional dive boat operator who had worked for years with Lloyd Bridges on his television series *Sea Hunt*. Mickey was more than a competent pilot; he was skilled at operating the boat for divers, putting his boat in and out of gear, idling, and gearing down to the speed of the diver. Just as important, he was eager to help Dave and realized that, given his speed and training, Dave had the potential to break the world record for the Catalina Channel. Mickey wanted to be part of that. For added safety, our father, a physician and a former U.S. Navy corpsman who had been on ships in the Pacific during World War II, went along to provide medical assistance if needed. Our mother and a friend, Helen Olsen, went along to feed and watch over Dave.

Dave swam for nine hours and fifty minutes, and Mickey and John helped him throughout the swim. With their support, Dave shattered the world record from Catalina Island to the California mainland.

A few years later, Mickey took me across on my second Catalina Channel swim, and with his support and Dave's coaching, I broke the world record from the mainland to the island.

Mickey's son, John Pitman, and Mickey's former partner, Greg Elliott, mentioned previously, are now escorting swimmers on their Catalina Channel swims. Both have had years of experience. Each man operates his own boat, and through the years, many swimmers have hired these pilots to escort them on their Catalina Channel swims.

You need to consider whether it's more important to hire one of the most experienced pilots for your swim, and have one day to attempt the swim, or find another pilot who will work with you before the swim and give you a number of options for the dates you will swim.

"If I were a well-resourced swimmer," L. Tadeus said, "I would assist a boat pilot and his crew in gaining the required experience outside the cabal of established pilots. It requires a significant amount of relationship and trust building. A pilot and crew can claim all the qualifications and experience in the world, but uneducated swimmers would lack the required knowledge to gauge their actual qualifications and experience. Swimmers who want to do this *must* become educated in seamanship and boat handling as well."

When planning my open water swims in remote parts of the world where swims have never been done, I've found it a challenge to locate a qualified pilot. If the person is intrigued with the idea of the swim, and eager to work with me and combine his local knowledge with mine, it's the start of a great team. One of the key things I do is set aside between five and ten days to make that connection; this gives me roughly two neap tides. I go through all the steps that I've written about in this book, draw upon my past experiences, discuss the project with my crew members who have been on past swims, and follow all the recommendations that the SEALs have given me for finding a qualified pilot, support boat, and crew.

There is a real advantage to having the pilot, crew members, and swimmer understand from their own experience what each person does during a swim. The SEALs realize that this creates some astounding synergy if the boat crews are trained in swimming (at least at a basic level) so they understand why swimmers do what they do and, more important, why they make the decisions they make midswim. It helps tremendously if swimmers understand how the pilot navigates the boat and supports the swimmer.

One of the SEALs' advantages is that every instructor has been through what all the trainees have been through. They also have had seamanship training. Trainees have *full* confidence in the instructor's ability to keep them safe and moving in the right direction, because they know the instructors have the safety piece under complete control.

You need to build trust with your pilot before the swim. Just because you've paid for a pilot to escort you, you cannot expect that he will make sure all the safety measures are in place. You have to make sure they are in place.

When you work with a new pilot, you take more responsibility for the outcome of your swim. One of the reasons David Yudovin has been so successful in swimming where no one has swum before is because he and his wife, Beth, are sailors and have their captain's licenses. They combine their knowledge of swimming with seamanship, and because of this, David has been able to accomplish swims that no one ever thought of attempting.

The SEALs would not plan a mission for a single day. They would not be driven by a sense of urgency, because they realize that this leads to accidents. They have backup plans and contingencies in place. They create what they describe as a "bump plan." If environmental conditions do not support an operation on a given day, they plan to roll the operation to a future date with the same plan, provided the target/opportunity is not a fleeting one.

You will want a bump plan so that you can make the swim another time if the conditions are not favorable.

MEETING WITH PILOTS BEFORE HIRING THEM

~ Before you attempt any swim, meet with your pilot and discuss the swim in great detail and create a basis of understanding.
~ A capable pilot will be skilled and be able to maneuver his boat.
~ He will be able to keep a swimmer as close to the escort boat as weather permits.

Two friends who swam the English Channel in different years had the same pilot. Both swimmers told me the same story: The pilot let each swimmer get up to a half mile (0.8 kilometers) ahead of the escort boat before he pulled alongside. They believed the pilot was trying to save fuel and money at the expense of their safety. Given the amount of shipping in the English Channel, the possibility of losing a swimmer to hypothermia, and other potential risks, a pilot should never permit a swimmer to be a half mile (0.8 kilometers) away from the escort boat.

If the wind is blowing engine fumes onto a swimmer, the pilot should be able to recognize that and reposition the boat so the swimmer is upwind of the fumes. Diesel fumes can make a swimmer sick and cause her to pass out.

INSPECT THE BOAT BEFORE YOU SWIM

I asked L. Tadeus: How do you know what size boat/ship is required for a channel swim? He said, "I wouldn't pick a ship until I knew at least three things: 1) what the average seas are like for that time of year; 2) what the international rules are for vessels regarding passengers; and 3) what the worst-case scenario would be for the mission/event.

"Then I would pick a vessel based on her sea-keeping capability; passenger capacity within international regulations and well above anticipated passenger load; and finally, the equipment on board for medical response, along with crew experience."

Before hiring a pilot for a channel swim, inspect the boat to make sure it is well maintained. Australian Des Redford taught me this. He was one of the world's top channel swimmers and among the most experienced English Channel swimmers. For years, he competed with Irish swimmer Kevin Murphy and British swimmer Michael Reed for the record for the most English Channel swims. Des was also the coach of some of Australia's top channel swimmers. He coached Susie Maroney, the twenty-two-year-old Australian swimmer who became the first person to swim (in a shark cage) from Cuba to Florida.

Des told me that on one English Channel swim, at the halfway point, the boat's engine broke. The pilot tried to fix the engine but couldn't get it started. Des did not want to climb out of the water or hang on to a rope, because under Channel Swimming Association rules, he would have been disqualified. Instead, he treaded water.

Eventually, he got cold and started swimming around the boat to get warm. About an hour later, the pilot finally fixed the problem, and Des started swimming again. This hour delay didn't just lengthen Des's time in the water; it made the entire swim more difficult because he missed the tide and had to fight for hours against strong current and headwinds.

The experience taught him to always check the boat out carefully and verify that it is in good shape. He knew in advance that the boat wasn't the best, and he had heard of boats breaking down on other channel swims. He said it is disappointing to be pulled out of a swim because of physical limitations, but it's worse when the boat breaks down when you are ready and you know you can complete the crossing.

BEFORE YOU BEGIN ANY CHANNEL SWIM

Evaluate the risks and work on mitigating them.

Shipping lanes in any channel can be dangerous, especially when fog moves in. In a twenty-four-hour time period, there are, on average, six hundred ships moving through the English Channel and eighty to a hundred ferry crossings between Dover, England, and Calais, France—one of the optimal landing points for the English Channel swim.

The ships—tankers, cargo ships, passenger ships, fishing and sailing boats, and leisure craft—all pose potential threats to swimmers. Tankers are enormous ships with a capacity that can range from several hundred tons to several hundred thousand tons. They operate in ocean channels, sailing through inland waters, across great lakes, and along deep rivers and canals. They move at a speed of up to nine knots through the English Channel. Some tankers are as long as football fields, and because of that size and momentum, they cannot stop for swimmers. The pilot's job is to monitor shipping traffic and check in with the UK Maritime and Coastguard Agency to figure out the speed of the ships and the swimmer's speed and determine if the swimmer can get safely through the shipping channels.

Sometimes tankers alter the course of swimmers. Stella Taylor, one of the great long-distance swimmers, grew up in England, became a nun, left the convent, and moved to Florida. She began training for the English Channel in her forties. In 1975 we met in Dover Harbor while we were waiting for neap tides and fair weather. Stella had bright blue eyes, short chlorine-bleached-blond hair, and a warm smile. She spoke with an eloquent British accent, and her eyes twinkled when she told me she was forty-three and people had told her she was too old to swim across the English Channel. I laughed and told her that I was fifteen years old and people had told me I was too young to swim across the English Channel. It didn't matter to either of us, because we had trained hard and we wanted to see what we could do.

We took off from Shakespeare Beach, near Dover, at about the same time, with different pilots. Throughout the swim, we thought of each other, and our pilots stayed in touch by radio and updated us on each other's progress. When I finished, my pilot radioed Stella's pilot, who said that Stella was still swimming strongly and that she had invited us to drop by for a cup of tea. It was so Stella.

Reg diverted our boat so we could meet her in the middle of the channel. She had been treading water for half an hour, waiting for a tanker to pass. When we reached her, she was bouncing in the tanker's wake just as it passed. The tanker's propellers churned up cold water, but Stella said it was refreshing. Her pilot tossed her a plastic water bottle filled with warm tea, and she said, "Will you join me for a cup of tea?"

While our boats pulled side by side and her pilot poured us tea in cups, Stella told us that she was feeling great and that she loved her pilot. He was doing a great job. The pilot handed us the steamy cups of tea, and we toasted her, and Stella said, "It's so lovely to be in the English Channel having tea with you." We laughed, and her pilot said that we couldn't keep her too long. He was afraid that she would cool down.

We watched her swim toward France. Her pilot was right beside her on the boat. We watched until they disappeared in the hazy horizon. When we arrived in Folkestone harbor, I kept thinking about Stella and wondered how she was doing. She swam for five more hours through rougher seas, with winds that gusted to thirty-five knots, but she made it to France, and that night when she returned to

Dover, we met and celebrated. Two years later, she would swim again and become the oldest woman to swim across the English Channel.

It is extremely important before a swim to look at the navigational chart that your pilot will use. Study the chart, so you have the course in mind. Work with your pilot to determine the best starting point. Often long swims are begun at night, when you cannot see the shore well or the barrier between you and the starting point. There are questions you need to ask: Are there rocks, reefs, underwater obstructions, pier pilings, or kelp beds? Are there fishing lines or buoys that you can become tangled in?

If the starting point is unfamiliar, it is worth getting to that area during the daytime and go by Zodiac, kayak, or small boat to see if there are any obstructions or other potential problems. The tide may be different when you begin your swim, higher or lower than when you first checked the starting point, and rocks that may be submerged during the day can pop out of the water at night.

If possible, go ashore in a Zodiac, with an experienced driver, and begin your swim from a sandy beach.

Once you have studied the starting point, based on your pilot's experience and your observations during the week before your swim, you will work with the pilot to determine the best course. And you will plan your swim route.

Remember to use the SEAL action plan for organizing your swim.

CONTACT THE U.S. COAST GUARD

Let the coast guard (USCG) know a few days in advance that you are planning a swim. You or your pilot need to give the coast guard the coordinates for the start of your swim, your proposed route and speed, and your estimated time of arrival and coordinates for that place. Often currents, tides, and winds will take you off course, but if something goes wrong during your swim, the coast guard will already have an idea of the course and may be able to render aid.

STAYING HEALTHY

There's nothing worse than training for a big swim and being worried about getting sick. While I love to travel, at times, sitting inside an aircraft cabin, hearing people coughing and sneezing, makes me feel like I am captive in a germ capsule. The problem is that the air inside the cabin is recycled and very dry and can cause dehydration. It is good to replace fluids as needed throughout the flight, but the dehydrating effect of the air can cause the nasal passages to dry out as well. The rhinovirus likes to attach to the dried nasal passages and infect the body. The last thing I want to do before a big swim is catch a cold.

It seemed to me that it might be possible to create a barrier to the virus with Aquaphor—a skin moisturizer like Vaseline that is usually used for cracked lips. I asked Dr. King if I could apply a tiny amount of Aquaphor inside my nose with a Q-tip. She agreed that it was worth trying, that Aquaphor is water soluble, though she did not recommend using Vaseline inside the nasal cavity because it is not water soluble.

On my flight from Buenos Aires to Ushuaia, Argentina, where I planned to train for my Antarctica swim, the idea was dramatically tested. A young man with a full-blown head and chest cold sat down beside me and started coughing hard. He didn't have a handkerchief. When he caught his breath, he apologized, and I told him there was no problem, but I was searching for a seat to move to, one that would put a great distance between us.

Unfortunately, the plane was full. The man with the head cold sat beside me for four hours and coughed the entire flight. Fortunately, I didn't catch his cold. My immune system might have been revved up because of my training—exercise stimulates the immune system—but I think the Aquaphor helped create a barrier to the germs.

BOATING SAFETY

One of the worst things that can happen on an open water swim is to have a swimmer run over by a boat. It is every swimmer's nightmare.

A few years ago a swimmer was in an open water race off Maui, Hawaii. He was a very strong swimmer and had been training up to six hours a day, but during the race, something went terribly wrong. The swimmer was having a great swim and then was hit by the safety boat. His right arm was amputated above the elbow. His left wrist and middle finger, thumb, and index finger were severed.

The news about this accident spread rapidly through the open water swimming community and everyone who heard about it wondered what went wrong.

No one seemed to have any answers, so I asked L. Tadeus of the SEALs how they would question the organizers to figure out what went wrong; put more safety measures in place next time; and prevent something like this from happening again. These are questions the SEALs would ask:

~ How long did it take emergency personnel to arrive on the scene?
~ Who responded to the mishap: lifeguards, EMTs, harbor patrol, USCG, other?
~ Was there an emergency action plan in place?
~ How long did it take law enforcement personnel to arrive on the scene?
~ Did the boater stop to help?
~ Did he take off?
~ Did he even notice he'd hit someone?

~ Why didn't the support crew put themselves between the oncoming boat and the swimmer(s)? (Were they protecting more than one swimmer?)

~ Did the support crew have any flags, day shapes, or lights indicating a swim was going on? (USCG requires that boaters adhere to the "rules of the road," regardless of licensing or competence.) Does anyone know if the swim was published in the *Notice to Mariners*?

~ Did the boater have a radio?

These questions go to a more specific level and let you see how important it is to think though every scenario when you are planning a swim.

SELECTING BOAT SUPPORT FOR AN ORGANIZED SWIM

The safety and success of any swim depends on the support pilots, their crews, and the maintenance of their boats. It takes a lot of meetings and discussions between event organizers and local officials, law enforcement, and U.S. Coast Guard to support a rough-water swim or triathlon event.

SEALs train for high-risk missions and make sure they have the support they need to ensure the safety of their group and complete their training mission. Often they have to organize and coordinate with different military and government groups to make sure everyone is working together.

When civilians are putting on an event, they should have the best boat support possible. The only way (currently) to regulate pilots is to require specific pilot/crew qualifications well in advance of events—and disallow unqualified support boats. There should be interaction with local law enforcement agencies and the U.S. Coast Guard. Ideally, there would also be a formal training program in place. In spite of all the things you do to support and organize a swim, there will be surprises, even for the pros.

L. Tadeus recounted a "nightmare dive" he witnessed not long ago:

> It was Friday night before the SEAL reunion that was marked by an uptick in maritime traffic in San Diego Bay. Needless to say, there were lots of drunken boaters on the water.
>
> We had thirty dive pairs in the water in Glorietta Bay, marked by well-lit buoys for safety. Rather than avoid them, several boaters (with passengers egging them on) took it upon themselves to approach the buoys. My very squared-away dive supervisor loudly ordered the support boats to ram any vessel approaching any dive buoy, and he communicated his intentions in no uncertain terms to other boaters. Our support boats were well lit—using red/white/red dive lights for night—but most civilians don't even know what this means.
>
> All were kept safe, but it required active and direct intervention by take-charge personnel on the surface. They even made contact with a couple of boats.
>
> The point of all this is: What would a given pilot do if a similar situation occurred during a competitive swim event? My guess is he would worry more about legal and financial liability than swimmer safety, so my recommendation is to have all pilots supporting a swim discuss safety procedures in advance with USCG and LLEA (local law enforcement). They would require authority that we possess outright and that they would not have without USCG and LLEA support.
>
> That is what support boats and supervisory personnel are supposed to do. I am guessing a significant lack of support contributed substantially to the swimmer losing a limb.

ORGANIZED SWIM CONSIDERATIONS

A few years ago, Sandy Field, a triathlete and open water swimming friend, competed in a race off Waikiki Beach in a field of five hundred swimmers. The swimmers set off in one large group. The problem came when they had to swim through a narrow opening between coral heads to reach open water.

Sandy was swimming at her pace when a male swimmer in his forties swam over her back and pushed her head underwater. She came up sputtering and said later that if she hadn't been a strong swimmer, she could have drowned. She shouted to the lifeguards and complained. At the end of the race, the meet organizers, the male swimmer, and Sandy discussed what had happened.

The meet organizer didn't do anything about it, which troubled Sandy, especially since she'd been asked to help organize the Orangeman Triathlon in Dana Point, California. She asked me what I thought. My first recommendation was to establish new rules for the new event and announce ahead of time that any swimmer who intentionally swam over another swimmer would be disqualified.

I spoke with L. Tadeus to find out how he would make the swim in the Orangeman Triathlon safer. He noted the problem with launching heats of five hundred swimmers at a time, which made it impossible to keep track of distressed swimmers and equally impossible to keep up with rule breakers. "Even if it were possible to find a distressed swimmer, how would you provide help in the middle of a group that huge, especially when there is a choke point?"

He recommended setting off no more than fifty swimmers at a time and making sure the safety observers at a choke point paid serious attention. The swimmers would be set off in thirty waves of fifty swimmers, staggered at thirty-second-to-one-minute intervals.

He would also have a shepherd's crook on hand for anyone who intentionally harmed another swimmer and police on standby. He would charge anyone who intentionally hurt another swimmer with assault, and create a blacklist like those used at casinos to keep out the undesirables. "The race director, in particular, has a responsibility to do something. Whatever he tolerates becomes the new rule. He has to think about organizational leadership here, not just his profit margin. Whoever runs the safest, most fair swims is going to profit the most. That's the one most new swimmers are going to flock to."

Sandy announced the new rule before the start of the Orangeman Triathlon: If anyone intentionally swam over or hurt another swimmer, the person would be disqualified.

After the race was over, the triathletes gave the organizers feedback: All of the swimmers had great swims, even people who did a triathlon for the first time. The meet organizers were thrilled that people said it was one of the most professionally organized triathlons. By redefining the rules for the swim and requiring the triathletes to conduct themselves in a sportsmanlike fashion, this swim may be the new example of the way the swim portion of the triathlon can be run and, in doing so, encourage a lot more people to participate in and enjoy the race.

Chapter 22

Swimmer's Utopia

Ways to Improve Training and Support and to Build Trust among Swimmers, Support Boats, and Physicians

On open water swims, whether you're doing short or long swims, it is important to have not only competent support but also people you can trust. Trust is a huge element in open water swimming. The pilot and crew's decisions affect the entire outcome of your swim.

What I've found during my open water swims is that the trust building begins for me when I first meet the potential pilot and crew. We sit down and discuss the swim together. Having done a lot of research beforehand, I am able to ask enough questions to stimulate a discussion and ideas for the swim.

Usually, I have spent weeks, months, or even years corresponding with a potential pilot and crew for an open water swim, so that by the time we meet, we have already developed a relationship and begun to build trust. Most pilots and crews are excited about supporting a swim and will volunteer to work with the swimmer during training sessions so they can see how the swimmer does and the swimmer can see how the pilot and crew work together. If something doesn't feel right about the pilot or crew, it probably isn't right, and you should consider another pilot. Your life may be in the pilot and crew's hands.

The SEALs work on developing an atmosphere of trust between the trainees and their instructors. This trust always begins at a very high level. The instructors remain professional in everything they do. Unprofessional behavior can and has damaged trust on occasion.

For the most part, the instructors have achieved what the trainees are striving to achieve, so the trainees look to the instructors as examples of how to get there. Not every instructor recognizes that immediately. Trust is further heightened through test gates, which are established standards that every trainee must meet to become a SEAL. Some of them are concrete standards; for example, in first phase, trainees must run four miles (6.4 kilometers) in thirty-two minutes on three of five runs. Another test gate, in second phase, might require a trainee to properly ditch and don his SCUBA equipment and give himself a dive check within five minutes—day or night. These test gates are crucibles that force trainees to reach beyond their perceived limits. If the trainees give themselves to the training and trust what the staff tells them, they achieve success. This trust building occurs very quickly.

As the sport of open water swimming continues to grow and people decide to take on greater challenges, I've wondered how we can emulate the SEALs. They have honed their skills, mentored one another, and have physicians and medical staff who support them. They have resources to help them train, plan missions, and achieve their objectives.

Chapter 23

Stewardship of the Waters

A few years ago, the Sheth Foundation invited me to speak about my swim in Antarctica to an eminent group of seven hundred people in Mumbai, India. As part of this journey, the hosts gave me the opportunity to explore Mumbai, the Arabian Sea, and the subcontinent. What I discovered was that Mumbai was one of the most energetic, diverse, and fascinating cities in the world, but also one of the ten most polluted cities in the world. The Arabian Sea, which flows slowly around Mumbai, is thick and opaque gray brown. When a heavy breeze sweeps over the sea's surface, the water smells of sewage, crude oil, chemicals, and rotting fish. Friends and I took a boat ride from Mumbai to Elephanta Island, a distance of 6.2 miles (10 kilometers), and the water never cleared.

At a reception after my talk, I met a tiny woman in her forties, dressed in a brilliant pink, turquoise, and yellow sari and wearing large dangling earrings. She had long dark brown hair and deep brown eyes. She was so excited because she had recently completed her doctorate in environmental studies. I asked her what she planned to do with her degree.

She said, "My goal is to clean up the Indian and Arabian seas."

I asked her with awe, "How do you plan to do that?"

She said with great confidence, "Through education."

Though it was mind-boggling to think that one person could make a difference, there have been individuals around the world who made a tremendous difference by informing people about their impact on the oceans and the life within them. Rachel Carson educated people about pesticides, their effects on the environment, and the need to manage them more wisely. Jacques Cousteau, a former French naval officer, explorer, ecologist, innovator, scientist, author, and researcher who codeveloped the Aqua-Lung, pioneered marine conservation. Through his films and photography, he opened new worlds within the ocean for people, and gave them an understanding of the fragility of this environment and the need to protect it.

More recently, Rivers Unlimited and the Sierra Club discovered that water quality standards were about to be lowered on the Ohio River. They needed to inform the local citizens about the damage this would do to the river and the economic fallout. They invited me to swim across the Ohio with local swimmers to make people aware of the plight of the river. The mayor of Cincinnati and the local media got behind the event, and more than seven thousand people living in Dayton, Kentucky, and Cincinnati, Ohio, contacted their local governmental officials, asking them to vote to maintain the water quality standards on the Ohio. The officials abided by their wishes.

Surfers often paddle for open water swimmers on their swims and have long been aware of the effects of water pollution, especially the effects of runoff from residential landscapes on their favorite surfing spots. They brought attention to the increases in sediments in the water and reduction in ocean water clarity. Surfers have seen the effects of runoff caused by fertilizers with increases in red tides, algae blooms, bacteria, and jellyfish populations.

Surfers, like swimmers, run into debris and garbage and have seen it choke and kill marine animals. They also understand that some pesticides used in residential landscapes poison fish and seep into our food chain. As a result, they started the Surfrider Foundation, a nonprofit environmental organization for the protection and enjoyment of the world's oceans, waves, and beaches for all people, through conservation, activism, research, and education. They have had a positive impact.

Often these environmental movements begin with the efforts of one person. Looking across the clear aqua waters of Monterey Bay today and watching adult sea otters with their young bobbing in thick kelp beds, observing pelicans and seagulls diving and plucking fish from the water, and seeing people swimming, kayaking, and scuba diving in the bay, I find it hard to imagine that just over one hundred years ago, Monterey Bay was nearly destroyed by overfishing sardines and abalone, that tons of fish guts and waste were dumped into the water daily, and that fumes from the scum floating on the waters were so bad that they turned lead-based paints black. Sea otters that inhabited the bay were hunted nearly to extinction.

It took only one person to realize that things could be changed. Dr. Julia Platt, a marine biologist from Pacific Grove, a neighboring town, decided to do something about it. She established a small marine refuge in Monterey Bay, prevented commercial fishing, and limited the amount of noncommercial extraction. She created a nursery "from where the tiny larvae may swim or be carried by currents to all points along the shore and become attached, grow up, and replace those taken."

By 1962 the bay was no longer contaminated by sardine offal, the abalone and sea urchins had increased in population, the sea otters had returned to Monterey Bay, and the kelp forests on which abalone and urchins grazed rebounded. Slowly, the bay has returned to its past glory. In 1984 Julie Packard, an environmentalist and visionary, gathered together a team of experts and, with their support and guidance, built Monterey Bay Aquarium in the "bones" of an old cannery. The Monterey aquarium is now a place of research and conservation.

Many of us are already doing simple things to tend the beach and waters. When we find glass or fishing lines on the beach, we carefully pick them up and throw them away so that swimmers, surfers, beachgoers, and wildlife won't be injured. When we see an abandoned hole in the sand dug by children who were having fun making sand castles and moats, we stop for a few moments to fill it in so that joggers or beach walkers won't fall in and injure themselves—as one friend did, who tore her ACL and needed surgery. We all have an impact on the waters and beaches, and we all can make a positive difference in maintaining their natural beauty.

As more people become involved in open water swimming and triathlons, my hope is that we can find ways to be stewards of our beaches and open waters. As you spend more time in the open water, you will find that you can feel the daily and seasonal rhythms of the lakes, rivers, and oceans. You will see wave and current patterns and changes. You will notice bird populations that migrate to and away from your shores. You will notice changes in the landscape and seascape, and through your journey, you will find friends who share the awe, wonder, and fun of swimming through worlds of water. For many of you, the open water will become a haven, a favorite place to visit, and many of you will discover that no matter where you are in the world, it will always be a place where you feel at home.

My goal was to share with you what I've learned from SEALs, scientists, physicians, and friends so that you can swim better and more safely in the open water. I hope you will love swimming beyond the waves and that being in the vast open water will inspire the great ideas and exciting dreams that you work toward and achieve.

Sources for Additional Information

INTRODUCTION

SEAL instruction:
www.sealswcc.com/navy-seals-buds-prep-docs.aspx

CHAPTER 1

Sports & Fitness Industry Association (formerly SGMA) study:
triathlon.competitor.com/2011/08/news/u-s-triathlon
-participation-reaches-2-3-million-in-2010_36864)

Triathlon Club of San Diego: www.triclubsandiego.org

CHAPTER 3

U.S. Masters Swimming: forums.usms.org/forum.php

Coney Island Brighton Beach Open Water Swimmers:
www.cibbows.org

YMCA Open Water Swim Training (YOWST): contact Tim
Treadwell at (631) 329-6884

East Hampton Volunteer Ocean Rescue:
www.easthamptonoceanrescue.org

Santa Barbara Swimming Association:
www.santabarbarachannelswim.org

Waikiki Swim Club: www.waikikiswimclub.org

Vision Quest Coaching: contact MarciaC944@aol.com

Tex Robertson Highland Lakes Challenge:
www.HighlandLakesChallenge.com

October Lake Travis Relay: www.laketravisrelay.com

American Swimming Association:
www.americanswimmingassociation.com

USA Triathlon: www.usatriathlon.org; to find a club, www.usa
triathlon.org/audience/clubs/club-listings/all-clubs-listings
.aspx; to find a coach, www.usatriathlon.org/audience/
coaching/find-a-coach.aspx

Revolution3: rev3tri.com

CHAPTER 5

Shotz Energy Gel: shotz1.com/products/shotz-energy-gel

Creatine: www.umm.edu/altmed/articles/creatine=000297.htm

CHAPTER 6

American Lifeguard Association: www.americanlifeguard.com

United States Lifesaving Association: www.usla.org

CHAPTER 13

Wilderness Medicine by Dr. Paul Auerbach: www.amazon
.com/Wilderness-Medicine-Enhanced-FeaturesAuerbach/
dp/1437716784

Safe Sea: www.bysafesea.com

U.S. Navy Diving Manual:
www.supsalv.org/pdf/DiveMan_rev6pdf

Hawaiian Lifeguard Association:
www.hawaiianlifeguardassociation.com

CHAPTER 14

Florida Museum of Natural History's International Shark Attack
File: www.flmnh.ufl.edu/fish/sharks/isaf/isaf.htm

CHAPTER 21

Catalina Channel Swimming Federation:
www.swimcatalina.com

HEAT AND COLD INJURY PREVENTION AND TREATMENT:

"Guidelines for Return to Work (Play) After Heat Illness: A Military Perspective," *Journal of Sports Rehabilitation*, 2007, 16.227–237, 2007, Human Kinetics, Inc., Francis G. O'Connor, Aaron D. Williams, Steve Bilvin, Yuval Heled, Patricia Deuster, and Scott D. Flinn.

"Prevention and Treatment of Heat Stress Injuries," *Navy Environmental Health Center Technical Manual NEHC-TM-OH-OEM 6260.6A*, June 2007, section C2.3.12, pp. 10–11, Navy Environmental Health Center Bureau of Medicine and Surgery.

"State of Alaska Cold Injuries Guidelines," Alaska Multi-level 2003 Version, Prepared by: Department of Health and Social Services Division of Public Health Section of Community Health and EMS, Box 110616, Juneau, AK 99811-0616, 907-465-3027, fax 907-465-4101, www.chems.alaska.gov.

SWIMMING TECHNIQUE:

Stroke work and drills for any age swimmer: *Fundamentals of Competitive Swimming for 8 and Under Swimmers Based on Breath Control, Balance, Sculling and Rhythm Skills*, Laura A. Cox, PDF (www.swimmingcoach.org/ecom/store/catalog/pdf/fundofcompswiminside.pdf).

SWIMMING EQUIPMENT MANUFACTURERS:

Adidas: www.adidas.com

Agonswim: www.agonswim.com

Arena: www.arenainternational.com

Dolfin: www.dolfinswimwear.com

Nike: www.nike.com

Speedo: www.speedousa.com

SWIMMING EQUIPMENT SUPPLIERS:

Competitive Aquatic Supply: www.casswimshop.com

J.D. Pence: www.jdpence.com

Swim Outlet: www.swimoutlet.com

MANUFACTURERS OF TRIATHLETE WET SUITS:

Aqua Sphere: www.aquasphereswim.com

Blue Seventy: www.blueseventy.com

Orca: www.orca.com/category/wetsuits

Profile Design: www.profile-design.com

TYR: www.tyr.com

Zoot: www.zootsports.com

O'Neill: www.oneill.com

MAP OF SAN PEDRO (CATALINA) CHANNEL:

www.charts.noaa.gov/OnLineViewer/18746.shtml

U.S. NAVY SEALS:

www.sealswcc.com/navy-seals-buds-prep-docs.aspx

Acknowledgments

A very special thank you to Vicky Wilson, my editor, who recognized the significance of the manual and helped shape it into a book that will help people to swim more safely in the open water and to enjoy the sport.

Thank you especially to Martha Kaplan, my agent, whose thoughtful comments enabled me to decide what needed to be included in the book and the best way to convey the material to the readers.

At Vintage, I would like to thank Anne Messitte, Stephen McNabb, Kathleen Cook, Beth Thomas, Claudia Martinez, Gabriele Wilson, Courtney Allison, Jocelyn Miller, Russell Perreault, Jennifer Marshall, and Charlotte Crowe, who contributed their expertise. They transformed the manuscript into a book and helped make sure it reaches its audience.

Many thanks to my friends Emmy Griffin, Raylene Molvius, Jay Molvius, Kathleen, Fessenden, Sandra Field, Deborah Ford, Dan Simonelli, Suzy Sullivan, Ed Schlenk, Jack Deshaies, Kathy Kusner, Vicky Guilloz, Sophie French, and Cindy Palin, all of whom offered invaluable suggestions.

Thank you to the scientists, physicians, lifeguards, and other experts who generously contributed their advice and knowledge to the book.

This book would not have been possible without the help and support of the U.S. Navy SEALs. With my great respect and deep appreciation, I thank you for giving me the opportunity to observe and learn from you, to adapt your methods, and to help open water swimmers.

Index